Breast Cancer and Breast Reconstruction

Edited by Luis Tejedor, Susana Gómez Modet, Lachezar Manchev and Arli Aditya Parikesit

Published in London, United Kingdom

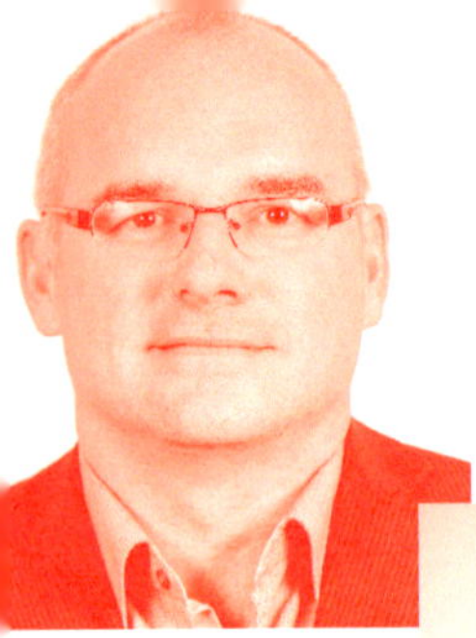
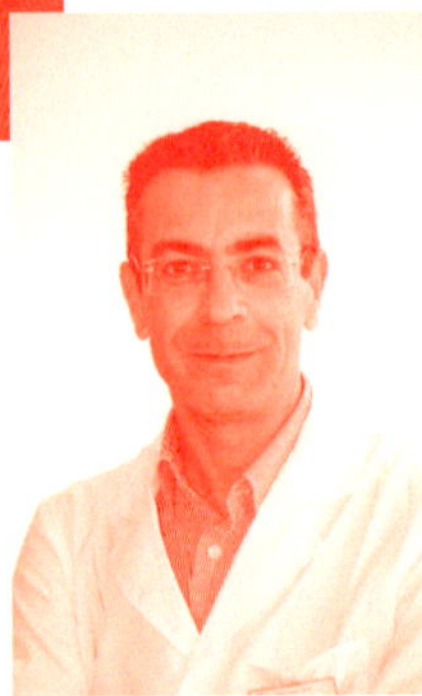
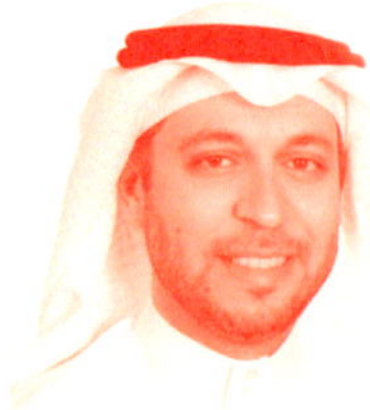
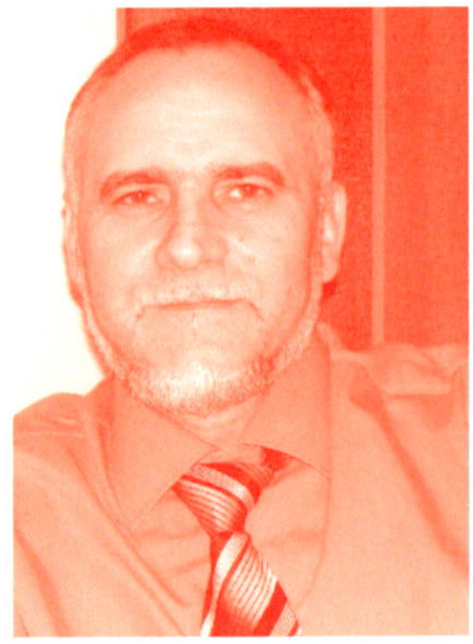
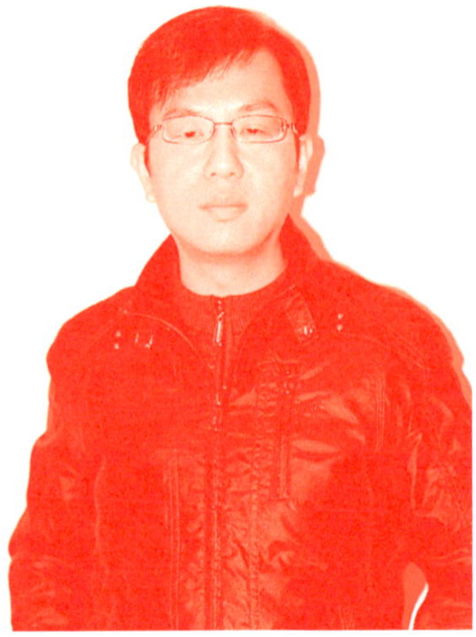
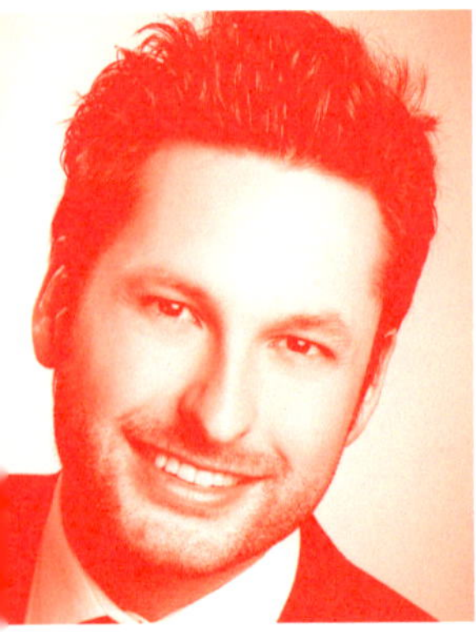
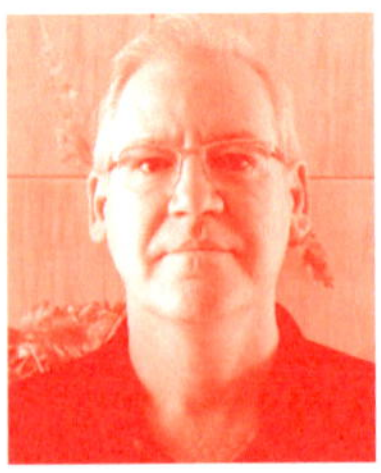

IntechOpen

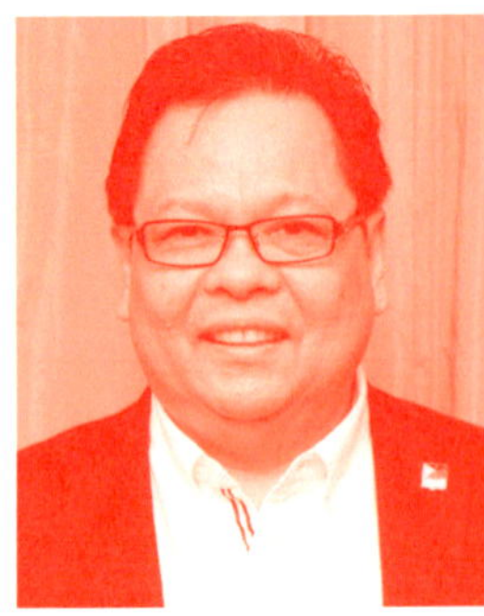
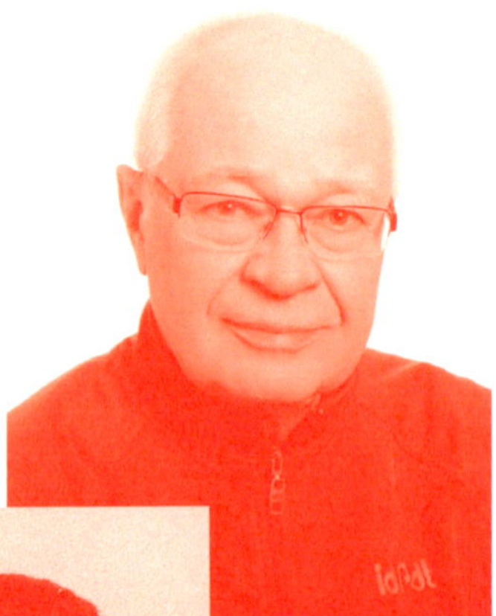
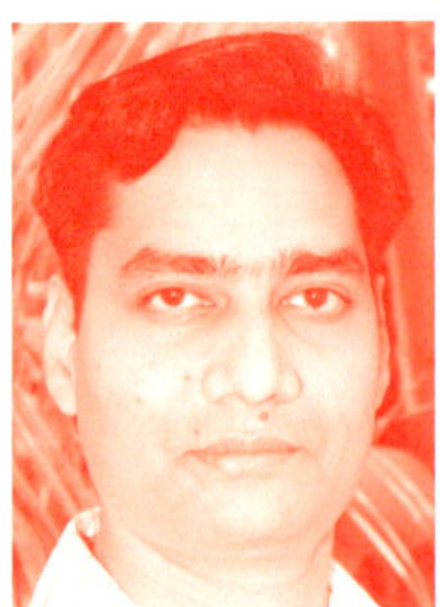
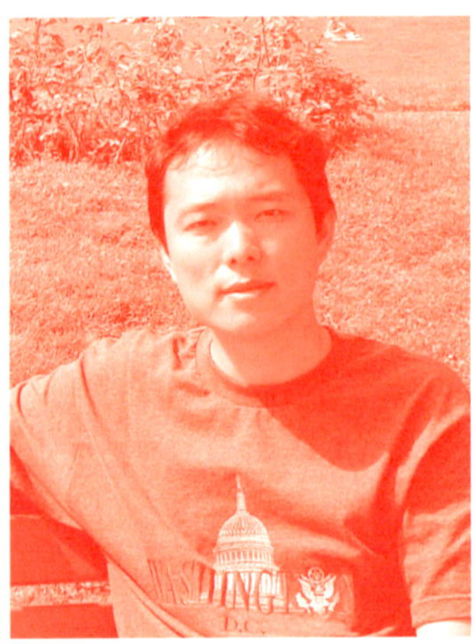
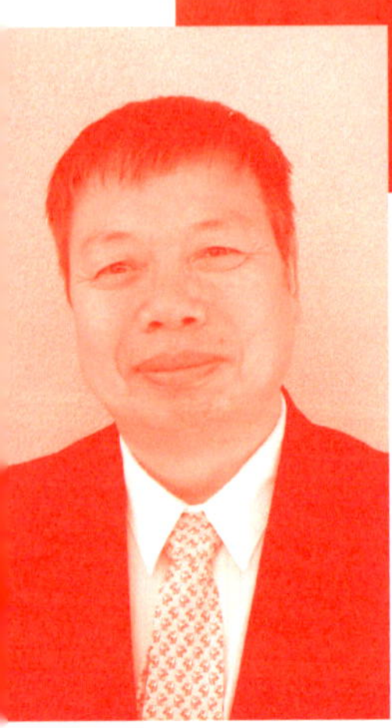
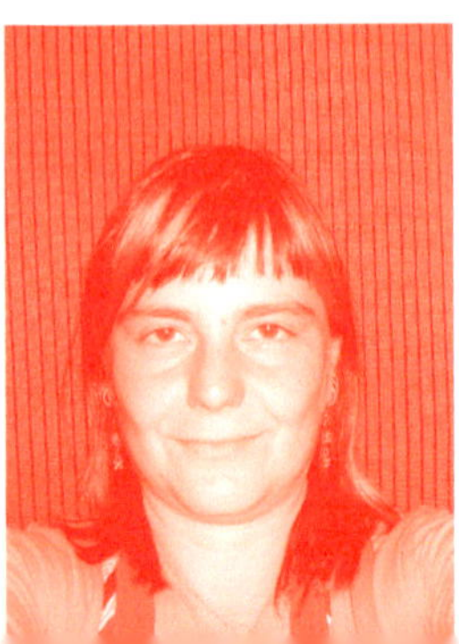

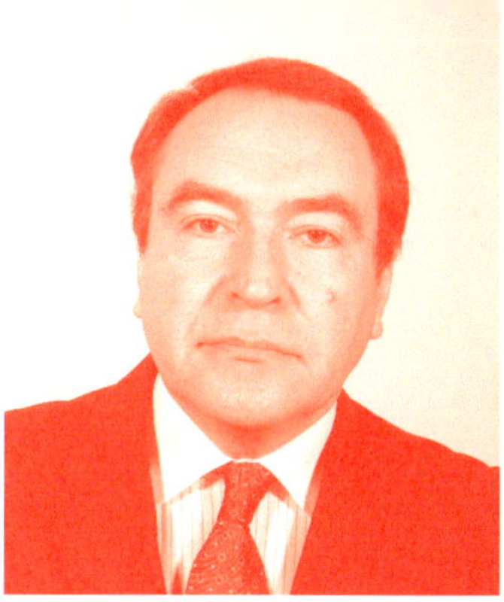
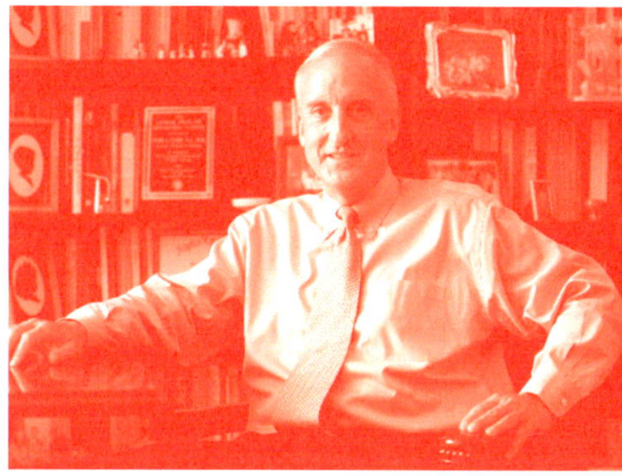
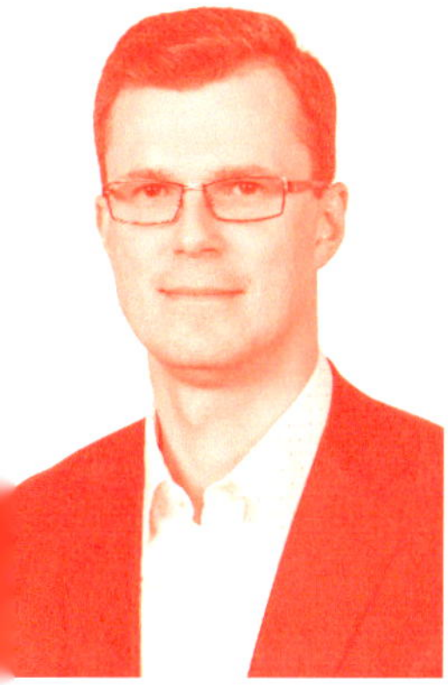
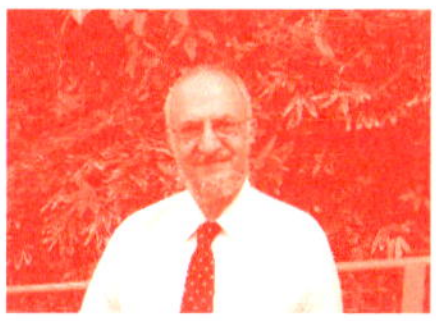
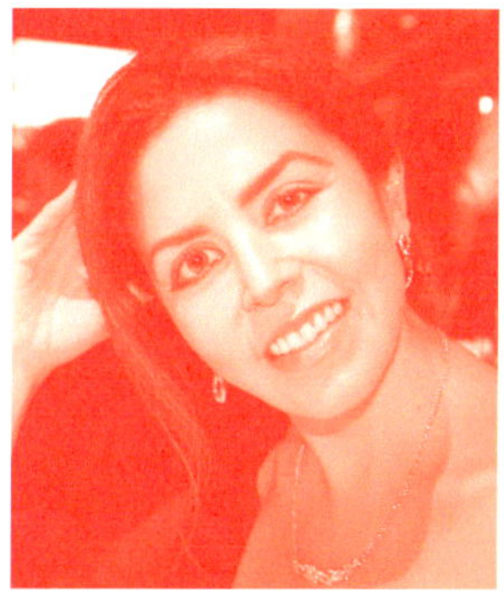

Supporting open minds since 2005

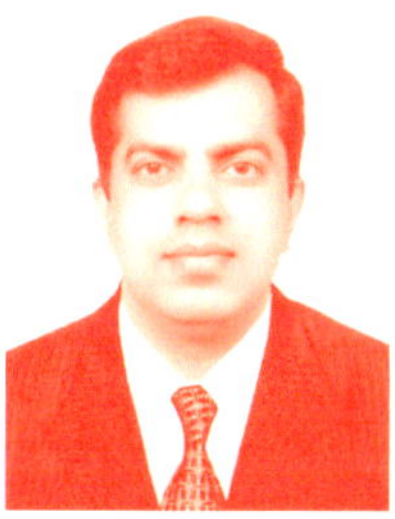
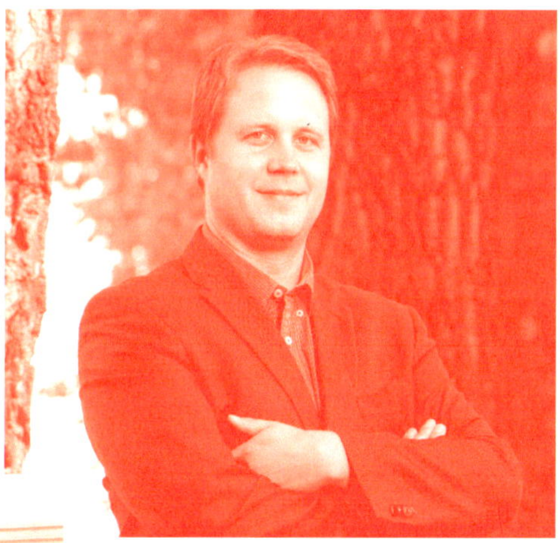
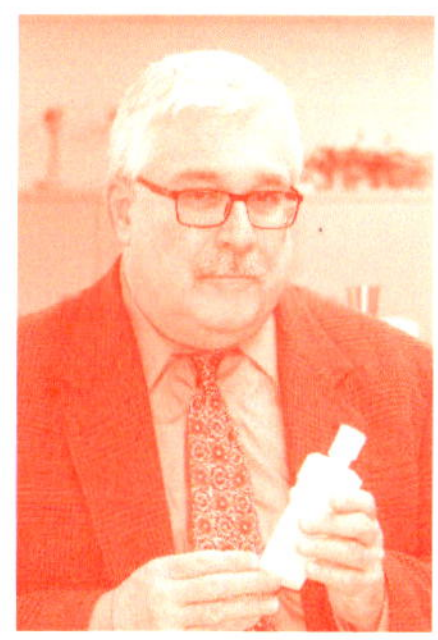
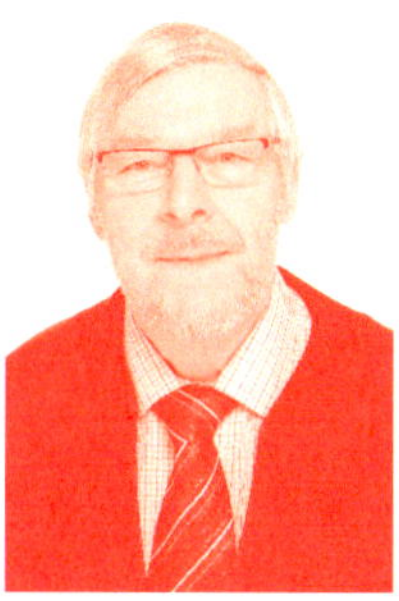
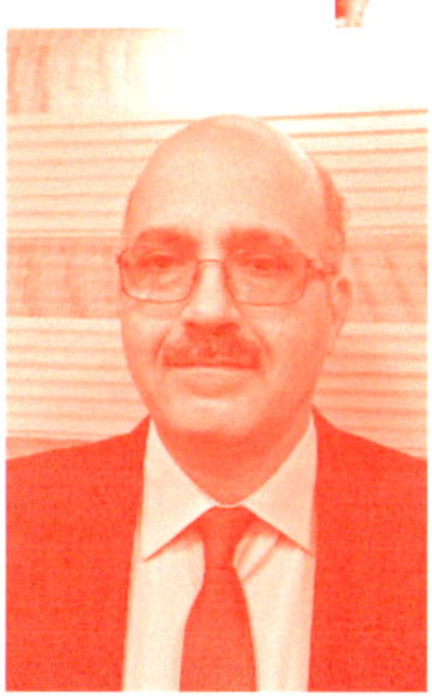
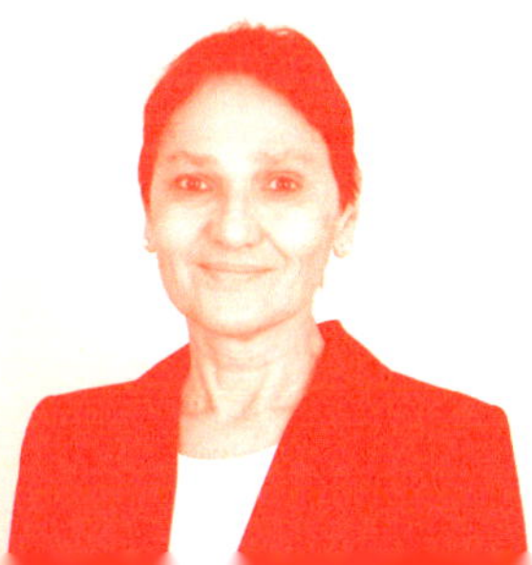
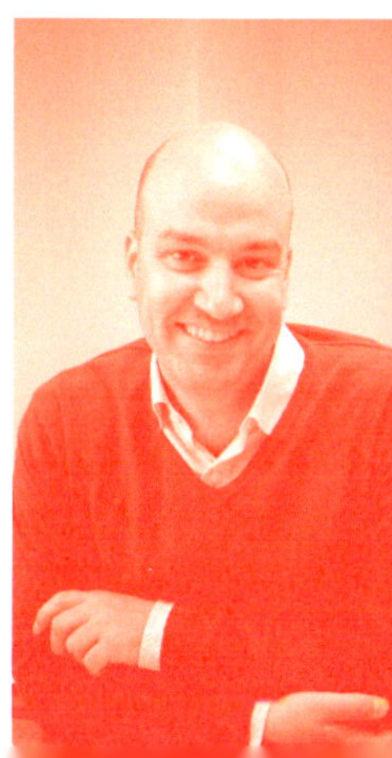

Breast Cancer and Breast Reconstruction
http://dx.doi.org/10.5772/intechopen.81453
Edited by Luis Tejedor, Susana Gómez Modet, Lachezar Manchev and Arli Aditya Parikesit

Contributors
Ercan Karacaoglu, Dung Nguyen, Justin Zelones, Suzanne Inchauste, Krishnamurthy S Murthy, David Atallah, Malak Moubarak, Abdallah Abdallah, Susana Gomez-Modet, Luis Tejedor, Anuja Antony, Ashley Woodfin, Alexander Karpov, Marina Korotkova, Gregory Shiferson, Elena Kotomina, Anwar Ebrahim, Naren Nath Basu, D. Gareth Evans, Maria Cristina Sini, Grazia Palomba, Giuseppe Palmieri, Antonio Cossu, Panagiotis Paliogiannis

First published in London, United Kingdom, 2020 by IntechOpen
IntechOpen is the global imprint of INTECHOPEN LIMITED, registered in England and Wales, registration number: 11086078, 7th floor, 10 Lower Thames Street, London, EC3R 6AF, United Kingdom
Printed in Croatia

British Library Cataloguing-in-Publication Data
A catalogue record for this book is available from the British Library

Additional hard and PDF copies can be obtained from orders@intechopen.com

Breast Cancer and Breast Reconstruction
Edited by Luis Tejedor, Susana Gómez Modet, Lachezar Manchev and Arli Aditya Parikesit
p. cm.
Print ISBN 978-1-78984-550-1
Online ISBN 978-1-78984-551-8
eBook (PDF) ISBN 978-1-83880-520-3

For EU product safety concerns:
IN TECH d.o.o., Prolaz Marije Krucifikse Kozulić 3, 51000 Rijeka, Croatia, info@intechopen.com or visit our website at intechopen.com.

Meet the editors

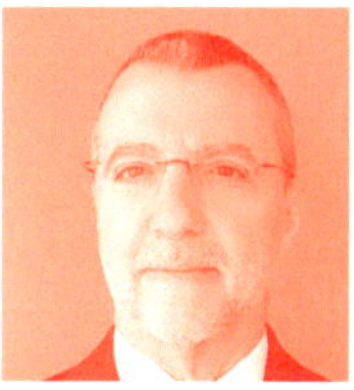

Luis Tejedor is a general surgeon with a particular interest in surgical oncology. His concerns led him to set up a complete and authoritative multidisciplinary Committee of Tumors in his hospital more than 25 years ago and to become a fellow of the European Board of Surgery Qualification in Surgical Oncology since its first announcement in 2003. In his clinical practice he has focused mainly on breast cancer, expanding his skills with masters, courses and attendances to breast cancer leading hospitals. He has been performing oncoplastic and reconstructive breast surgery for more than 20 years in the Breast Unit of his National Health System Hospital.

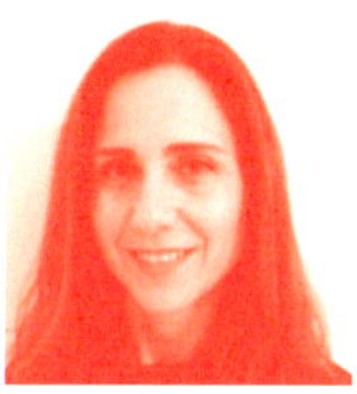

Susana Gómez Modet is a medical doctor who graduated from the University of Cádiz Medicine School, Spain, in 2000. She was trained as a General Surgeon in Málaga, Virgen de la Victoria Hospital from 2002 to 2007. Since then she has worked as a general surgeon, mainly in the Oncology Breast Surgery at Punta Europa Hospital, Algeciras, Cádiz, Spain. She completed her training in Senology with other academic titles: a Masters in Breast Diseases and Senology from the Barcelona University and an Expert Course in Oncoplastic and Reconstructive Surgery of the Breast. She is currently part of the Breast Unit and of the Committee of Breast Cancer in Punta Europa Hospital.

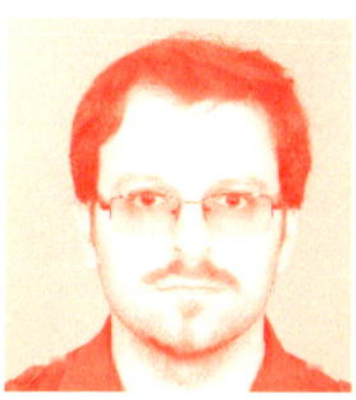

Associate Professor Lachezar Ivanov Manchev (MD, PhD) graduated in medicine from the Medical Faculty, Trakia University, Stara Zagora in 2010. Since 2010, he has worked as a radiologist in the Department of Diagnostic Imaging at the University Hospital, Stara Zagora. Between 2013 and 2018, he was assistant professor in the Department of Radiology in the Medical Faculty, Trakia Universtity, Stara Zagora. Since 2018, he has been an associate professor in Radiology at the same university. In his practice, he presents lectures and tutorials in Bulgarian to medical, nursing, midwifery and rehabilitation students, in subject areas including X-ray, CT, MRI, angiography, mammography, ultrasound and DSG. Dr Manchev also delivers lectures and tutorials in English to medical students from the United Kingdom and the Republic of Ireland. Since 2016, he works as a part-time lecturer for the Faculty of Public Health and Health Care, University Professor Doctor Asen Zlatarov, Burgas, Bulgaria.

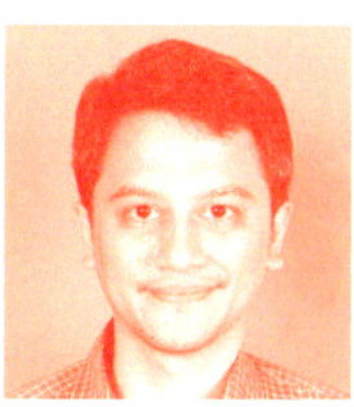

Dr Arli Aditya Parikesit is the Head of the Bioinformatics Department at i3L. He finished his bachelor and master degrees, both in Chemistry, from the University of Indonesia. In order to pursue his degree in Bioinformatics, he accepted a DAAD (German Academic Exchange Service) fellowship to conduct his doctorate research with the Bioinformatics Group, Faculty of Informatics and Mathematics, University of Leipzig, Germany. His doctoral research is focused on the utilization of modern protein domain annotation techniques to the three domains of life. In addition, Dr Arli is also an expert on immunoinformatics, in silico drug design, and in silico transcriptomics.

Contents

Preface XI

Section 1
Oncologic Issues 1

Chapter 1 3
Electrical Impedance Mammography: Screening and Basic Principles
by Alexander Karpov, Marina Korotkova, Gregory Shiferson and Elena Kotomina

Chapter 2 23
Detection of Breast Cancer in Mammograms through a New Features Technique
by Anwar Yahy Ebrahim

Chapter 3 33
Breast Cancer and *BRCA1* and *BRCA2* Pathogenic Variants
by Naren Basu and D. Gareth Evans

Chapter 4 49
Epidemiology and Genetic Susceptibility of Breast and Ovarian Cancer in Sardinian Population
by Grazia Palomba, Giuseppe Palmieri, Antonio Cossu, Panagiotis Paliogiannis and Maria Cristina Sini

Chapter 5 65
Genetic Mutation Carriers: Special Considerations for Their Influence on a Modern Breast Reconstruction Practice
by Ashley A. Woodfin and Anuja K. Antony

Section 2
Breast Conservative Surgery: Oncoplasties 79

Chapter 6 81
Oncoplastic Surgery in Breast Cancer
by Atallah David, Moubarak Malak and Abdallah Abdallah

Section 3
Breast Reconstruction **99**

Chapter 7 **101**
Breast Reconstruction with TRAM Flap
by Ercan Karacaoglu

Chapter 8 **111**
Immediate Breast Reconstruction with Free Autologous Tissue Transfer
by Justin Zelones, Suzanne Inchauste and Dung Nguyen

Chapter 9 **141**
Synthetic Mesh in Immediate Breast Reconstruction
by Susana Gómez-Modet and Luis Tejedor

Chapter 10 **161**
L-Shaped Nipple Reconstruction: A Novel Technique to Improve Patient Satisfaction Outcomes
by Krishnamurthy Sreedhar Murthy

Preface

Quoting one of the great masters in breast reconstruction, Scott L Spear, "the primary mission of a physician is to help his or her patients; the higher mission of a medical textbook is to help other physicians help even more patients". With this target in mind, this book has been devised to collect some recent data on a worldwide health problem. Breast cancer constitutes a notable problem in women's health and therefore a burdensome weight for society. Attempts to widen the knowledge on this disease, either at its preclinical (genetics) or clinical phase (diagnosis, treatment) are always welcome since they may lead to a decrease in the suffering (pain, physical dysfunctions, disfiguration, depression and so on) and a lengthening in survival of the patients. Authors have been busy to provide valuable information in these areas, so it is my hope that this book contributes in part to the mission expressed above.

Luis Tejedor MD, FACS, FEBS-SO
Chairman of General Surgery Service,
Hospital Punta de Europa,
Algeciras, Spain

Dr. Susana Gómez Modet
Cádiz University,
Spain

Lachezar Manchev, PhD
Associate Professor,
Trakia University,
Stara Zagora, Bulgaria

Dr.rer.nat Arli Aditya Parikesit
Department of Bioinformatics,
Indonesia International Institute for Life Sciences,
Jakarta, Indonesia

Section 1

Oncologic Issues

Chapter 1

Electrical Impedance Mammography: Screening and Basic Principles

Alexander Karpov, Marina Korotkova, Gregory Shiferson and Elena Kotomina

Abstract

Nowadays, screening uses the method of X-ray mammography for the early diagnosis of breast cancer. However, as a screening method, X-ray mammography has its limitations, such as age, periodicity of screening, 'dense' mammary gland and dynamic survey (repeated radiation). In order to overpass these limitations, more advanced alternative methods of breast examination should be used, which would be as effective as the 'golden standard.' Characteristics of electroimpedance diagnostics are given. The aim of screening is to detect breast cancer including early breast cancer (tumor size below 1 cm) and to form a survey of high-risk group. In order to reach these aims, the following actions need to be undertaken: search for areas with anomalous conductivity, detection of distorted mammographic scheme and evaluation of age-related electrical conductivity. The application of a scale for age-related breast conductivity with defined percentile limits allows to organize a survey group. Electrical properties of a cancerous tumor differ significantly from those of the surrounding tissues. Statistics of anomalous conductivity in cases of breast cancer is given. The disease development connected with the destruction of epithelial basement membrane is linked with various phenomena occurring in the tumor and the surrounding tissues. Statistics of disrupted mammographic scheme in cases of cancer is given.

Keywords: electroimpedance mammography, breast cancer, survey group, mammary gland structure, age-related electrical conductivity, anomalous conductivity, distorted mammographic scheme

1. Introduction: problems of breast cancer screening

In 1968 James Maxwell Glover Wilson and Gunnar Jungner supported by the World Health Organization published a research named [1]. In 1972 the American Cancer Society together with the National Cancer Institute developed the Breast Cancer Detection Demonstration Project, aimed to perform X-ray mammography breast cancer screening for more than quarter of a million of American women.

Since then, X-ray mammography has become not only the main screening method but also the 'gold' standard in diagnostics. It is important to distinguish the difference between screening tests and early diagnostics. Early diagnostics implies early detection of tumors in patients with symptoms. Screening test means early detection of tumors in patients without symptoms [2]. Nowadays, screening uses X-ray mammography as the method of early diagnostics of breast cancer. However, used as a screening method, X-ray mammography has its limitations and drawbacks. We'll name some problems of the main screening method.

Age. Women aged below 40 usually do not undergo breast cancer screening since sensitivity of mammography is low in this population due to the high density of breast tissue [3]. It was discovered that mammographic screening under the age of 50 is not only less effective than in the elder age but is also related to higher radiation risks [4]. Shifting of screening to the age range below 40 is undesirable since it will lead to the increase of patients' radiation exposure. Age limitations for X-ray mammography are closely related to breast cancer morbidity.

Morbidity. According to the data of the Health and Social Care Information Centre [5], despite screening programs, breast cancer morbidity does not decrease; it remained on the same level for all age groups for 10 years since 2004–2005 till 2014–2015 (**Table 1**). For the sake of solving the problem of morbidity, it would seem only natural to shift the screening framework down along the age scale. But age limitations do not allow for that.

Operational characteristics (sensitivity and specificity). Screening survey is a survey with low prevalence. As a rule, a low-prevalence survey is a preventive checkup. Screening survey is characterized by unrestricted sampling, usually estimated in many thousands, by low prevalence, standardized procedure, significant predominance of healthy patients over patients with pathologies, impossibility to use a reference method and histological verification of diagnosis due to a large number of healthy patients, significant predominance of early stage of disease among the affected patients and impossibility to apply operational characteristics, i.e. sensitivity and specificity. It is impossible to get operational characteristics and incidence data from the screening survey data. Operational characteristics can be received from the examination of patients with symptoms.

Table 2 shows operational characteristics of X-ray mammography received during a 6-year period from a large group of patients with symptoms [6].

Sensitivity of X-ray mammography used for breast cancer diagnostics above 80%, which would satisfy screening requirements, is observed only in the 70–79, 80–89 and 90+ age groups.

Breast density. Breast cancer is often similar to X-ray density of fibroglandular tissue, which makes it difficult to distinguish these tissue types due to the masking effect of dense glandular tissue [7]. It explains the unreliability of X-ray mammography for cancer diagnostics in women with high-density glandular parenchyma, with fibrocystic disease. Women with high mammographic density have higher

Women with cancer detected (rate per 1,000 women screened) by age group

England, 2004-05 to 2014-15 — rates

Age group	2004-05	2005-06	2006-07	2007-08	2008-09	2009-10	2010-11	2011-12	2012-13	2013-14	2014-15
50-54	6.4	6.3	6.4	6.3	6.3	6.3	6.2	6.6	6.7	7.0	6.7
55-59	6.7	6.8	6.7	6.7	6.5	6.2	6.0	6.3	6.6	6.5	6.7
60-64	8.9	8.8	8.5	8.5	8.6	8.6	8.4	8.6	8.9	9.0	8.9
65-70	11.7	11.6	11.3	11.2	10.2	10.1	10.1	10.4	10.3	11.1	11.0
Over 70	16.0	17.0	16.4	15.5	14.5	15.4	14.7	13.9	14.6	15.6	14.8

Source: KC62 (Parts 1 and 3, Table T) Health and Social Care Information Centre - see also Table 9a in Data Tables.

Table 1.
Women with cancer detected by age group.

Diagnostic procedure	Age group (years)	Number of women	Prevalence of breast cancer (%)	Sensitivity (%)	Specificity (%)	ROC area
Mammography	<30	15[a]	40.0	83.3	88.9	0.86
	30–39	1909	4.4	47.6	99.9	0.74
	40–49	4238	5.7	51.2	99.8	0.76
	50–59	2301	8.6	55.6	99.9	0.78
	60–69	1170	14.0	68.9	99.8	0.84
	70–79	925	27.0	79.8	99.3	0.90
	80–89	389	43.0	86.1	97.3	0.92
	90+	56	54.0	86.7	92.3	0.90
	Overall	11003	10.0	66.6	99.7	0.83

ROC, receiver operating curve.
[a]Data should be interpreted with caution as extremely small numbers of patients.

The British Journal of Radiology, April 2012

Table 2.
The number of patients attending the symptomatic breast clinic, by age and final diagnosis of either having breast cancer or not having breast cancer.

risk of breast cancer occurrence [8]. It has been proved that high mammographic density can be related to quadruple increase of breast cancer risk [9, 10].

Formation of survey or risk group. According to the definition of the World Health Organization, 'there should be a recognizable latent or early symptomatic stage. The natural history of the condition, including the early stage, should be adequately understood.' With the help of screening, it becomes possible to form breast cancer risk groups. Since ductal carcinoma takes origin from epithelial cells, areas with fibroglandular tissues and large amount of cells are highly susceptible to the increased epithelial proliferation [11]. It is the quantitative estimation of the state of fibroglandular tissue that should be used as the selection criterion allowing to differentiate the norm and the pathology. Patients with the amount of fibroglandular tissue abnormal for their age should become a part of the surveillance group. The existing screening methods do not allow to form breast cancer surveillance groups.

Repetitive examinations. Screening is a dynamic process. Recall of a patient for the screening program may cause anxiety or serious worries about potential illness, the so-called Ulysses syndrome, and lead to repeated radiation exposure [12]. In this connection, it is sensible to use safe screening methods that allow for multiple repetitive examinations. Frequency of examinations especially among high-risk group patients and in cases of hormone replacement therapy is chosen on an individual basis depending on the pathology detected.

Radiation exposure. Glandular tissue in the breast is most susceptible to radiation exposure compared to fat, skin and areola since immature cells are more vulnerable to ionizing radiation exposure [13]. And since ductal carcinoma takes origin from epithelial cells, it leaves one perplexed why X-ray mammography is used in breast cancer screening programs. Mammography has increased risks of radiation-induced breast cancer. Supposedly, low radiation dose is riskier than higher radiation dose [14, 15].

Rupture risk. The mammography procedure carries a risk of rupture of encapsulated cancer tumor, which may occur during the compression of breast tissue, and it may lead to metastases. Modern mammography equipment uses 42 pounds of pressure [16]. It may suffice for the disintegration of capsule and formation of metastases.

Mammography technique. According to the criteria of disease screening, the diagnostic method should be accessible and acceptable for the population [1]. Mammography technique can be evaluated through the analysis of the dose applied, the quality and size of the ray and the specific compression of breast. It has been established that the radiation dose and growth of breast cancer incidence are related [13]. Direct calculations of radiation dose (mGy) for a specific mammary gland are impossible. The difficulty lies in the knowledge of the structure of a specific mammary gland, which is necessary for the calculation of the conversion ratio. For this reason, an average dose is used, which depends on the thickness of the breast. In modern mammographs, the exposition is selected automatically based on the thickness of the compressed breast. Specific compression of the breast is the baseline for a good-quality image. Errors that may occur in the calculation of breast thickness during the compression of breast are related to the compression panel that may get bended and deformed.

These data show the necessity to implement additional effective screening programs for young women including screening with the application of alternative technology in order to lengthen the preclinical detection stage, which would lead to the decrease of breast cancer mortality rate [17]. In order to overcome the existing limitations, it is necessary to use modern alternative methods of breast examination that would be equal to the 'gold' standard in its effectiveness. Electrical impedance mammography is a diagnostic method satisfying the criteria set by the World Health Organization for screening for diseases. MEIK v.5.6, electrical impedance mammograph developed and manufactured by PKF 'Sim-technika,' Russia, uses advanced technologies of imaging and processing of electrical impedance images of breast. It is a noninvasive technology of image creation, it uses 3D-tomography system, it is a form of 'soft-field' tomography, it applies 'non-local' method of tomographic image creation and cross-sectional approach to data collection, it uses back-projection method as the algorithm of image reconstruction, and finally it allows to receive quantitative diagnostic information. The electrical properties of biological tissue as of colloid-dispersed system in an alternating electric field depend on the concentration and behavior of the chemical components of the tissue. The electric properties of a tumor differ significantly from those of the surrounding tissues. The aim of screening is to detect breast cancer including early breast cancer (tumor size below 1 cm) and to form a survey or high-risk group. In order to reach these aims, the following actions need to be undertaken: search for areas with abnormal conductivity, detection of distorted mammographic scheme and evaluation of age-related electrical conductivity.

2. Formation of survey group

Breast cancer risk factors. A notion exists of risk factors for breast cancer development. High breast density is one of the strongest risk factors for breast cancer development. Many of the stated risk factors for breast cancer influence breast density in the long run through hormones. Women with high breast density have higher concentration of estrogen in blood serum than women with lower breast density, and the risk of breast cancer for them is twice as high compared to the low level of circulating estrogens [18]. For women with extremely high breast density, the relative risk of breast cancer is four to eight times higher than high breast density or about two times higher than medium breast density [19]. Relative risk of breast cancer for women with extremely high breast density is 6.0 [with 95% confidence interval, 2.8–12.9], and it is the third risk factor after the patient's sex and age [20]. Search for risk factors, diagnostics and preventive measures for high breast density forms a new field of research.

High breast density. Breast density is inversely proportional to the content of adipose tissue and directly proportional to the content of epithelial and fibrous tissue [21]. With advancing age, breast density decreases, and the breast tissue 'ages' [21]. Serial mammography showed that the initial breast density influences the change of density through life: age-related decrease of high density is stronger than the density decrease in cases of lower density [22]. It was found that there exists a relation between high breast density and hormonal status. The specific features of reproductive anamnesis, menstruation anamnesis, menopausal status, excessive weight and exogenous and endogenous hormones influence breast density. Women with high breast density have higher concentration of estrogen in blood serum than women with lower breast density. Estrogen replacement therapy in pre- and postmenopausal period increases breast density [23–25]. Therefore, 'breast density' marker has higher potential as to being used for the prevention of breast cancer [26].

Methods of breast density estimation. Detecting women with high density of breast is the primary objective for screenings. Today there is no set 'gold' standard for the estimation of breast density. There are several methods for the assessment of breast density. Visual methods are based on the qualitative analysis of breast parenchyma, such as in Wolf's, Tabàr's, Boyde's and BI-RADS classifications. The aim of semiautomatic estimation is to measure breast density. There exist automated systems for the estimation of the area of breast density. Volumetric methods allow to evaluate the actual volume of fibroglandular tissue. It should be noted that various methods of breast density measurement use only X-ray systems. There is a sharp need for additional screening of women with high breast density [27]. Due to the growing interest toward estimation of breast density, new diagnostic methods appear.

Electrical impedance estimation of breast structure. Biological tissue is presented as a colloidal dispersion system. The structure of breast has a number of tissues that fulfill different functions (epithelial tissues, connective tissues, nervous tissue, blood and lymph) and fill the anatomical structures. The electrical properties of tissues are the direct consequence of the tissue structure. The electrical impedance mammograph MEIK v.5.6. with current force 0.5 mA and frequency of 50 kHz allows to evaluate breast structure. The fundamental difference of electrical impedance scanning from other tomography methods is that besides visual evaluation of the image, the electrical impedance mammography provides quantitative information, i.e. the numerical estimation of its anatomical and histological structure. This unique information is used for diagnostic purposes. All other factors equal, the electrical conductivity will depend on the concentration of ions and the amount of cellular elements, and it will decrease as the concentration grows [28]. The electrical conductivity index [IC], which is received during electric impedance scanning, is a quantitative characteristic of breast structure. Low index of electrical conductivity is typical for the breast containing a large amount of cellular elements and high concentration of ions, which corresponds to acinar-ductal type of breast structure. High electrical conductivity index is typical for the breast containing a large amount of fat lobules and connective tissue and low concentration of ions, which corresponds to amorphous structure of the breast. One thousand six hundred thirty-two processed images received from electromammographic examinations of healthy women helped to evaluate, percentile method applied, the structure of breast from the point of view of electrical impedance mammography. **Table 3** shows percentile limits for different types of breast structure in electrical impedance mammography.

Therefore, the electrical conductivity index can be used for the evaluation of breast structure from the point of view of electrical impedance mammography. It is a known fact that the structure of breast defines the breast density. For this reason, the defined ranges of electrical conductivity correspond to different types of 'density' of breast. **Table 4** shows the structure of the breast according to the electrical impedance mammography and types of density according to American College of Radiology [ACR] classification. 'Dense' breast, i.e. the so-called acinar-ductal type, is characterized by low electrical conductivity index. High electrical conductivity index is common for amorphous type of breast [consisting mostly of adipose and connective tissue]. The image shows examples of electrical impedance mammograms of patients from different age groups with different structure of breast: a 25-year-old patient with acinar-ductal type (**Figure 1**) and extreme breast density and 63-year-old patient with amorphous structure and low breast density (**Figure 2**).

Definition	Electrical conductivity	Percentile limits
Amorphous structure	More than 0.66	>90‰
Mixed type with amorphous component prevailing	0.57–0.65	75–90‰
Mixed type	0.30–0.56	25–75‰
Mixed type with acinar-ductal component prevailing	0.22–0.29	10–25‰
Acinar-ductal type prevailing	Less than 0.22	<10‰

Table 3.
Percentile limits for different types of breast structure in electrical impedance mammography.

	EIM classification	Electric conductivity	*ACR classification*
Type Ia	Amorphous	above 0,66	Predominantly fat, parenchyma below 25%
Type Ib	Mixed with the predominance of the amorphous component	0,57 – 0,65	
Type II	Mixed	0,30 – 0,56	Fat with some fibroglandular tissue, parenchyma between 25% and 50%
Type III	Mixed with the predominance of the ductal component, high density of the ductal component	0,22 – 0,29	Heterogeneously dense, parenchyma 50-75%
Type IV	Ductal, extremely high density of the ductal component	below 0,22	Extremely dense, parenchyma 75-100%

Table 4.
The structure of the breast according to electrical impedance mammography and types of density according to the American College of Radiology [ACR] classification.

On the **Figure 2** you can find examples of electrical impedance mammograms of the same age group but with different breast structure: 36-year-old patient with acinar-ductal type and high tissue density and 34-year-old patient with amorphous structure and low tissue density (**Figure 2**). In order to form a survey group, it is necessary to determine not only the breast structure but also the correspondence between the structure type and age-related electrical conductivity of the breast.

Electrical impedance evaluation of age-related electrical conductivity of the breast. The application of percentile method for the electrical impedance mammograms of healthy women in the following age ranges, <20, 20–29, 30–39, 40–49, 50–59, 60–69 and >70 years old, allowed to evaluate age-related electrical conductivity of the breast from the point of view of electrical impedance mammography. For each age group, the 5th, 50th and 95th percentile limits of electrical conductivity were calculated. The data can be represented in the form of percentile curves of

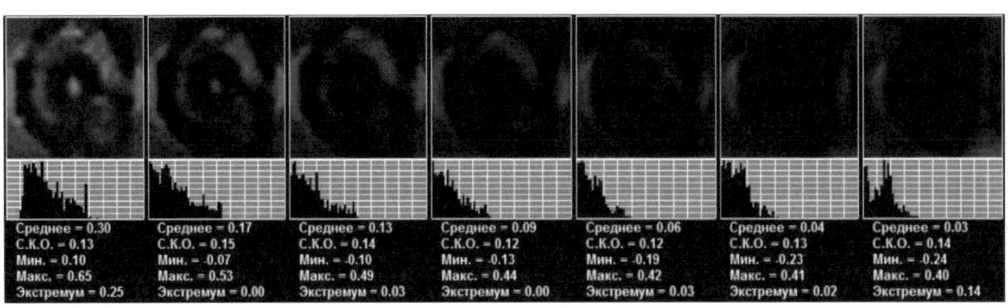

Figure 1.
Type IV (ACR IV). Acinar-ductal type. Extreme tissue density.

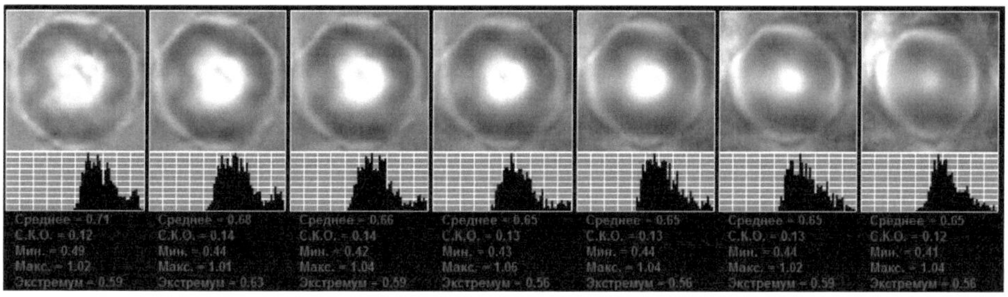

Figure 2.
Type I (ACR I). Amorphous type. Low tissue density.

Age range,years	5 percentile	50 percentile	95 percentile
20-29	0,18	0,28	0,44
30-39	0,16	0,40	0,53
40-49	0,22	0,51	0,63
50-59	0,32	0,58	0,72
60-69	0,43	0,57	0,78
over 70	0,50	0,57	0,64

Table 5.
Diagnostic table of age-related electrical conductivity of breast.

age-related electrical conductivity and in the form of a diagnostic table (**Table 5**). In accordance with the suggested estimations, the values in the 1st percentile corridor [below the 5th percentile] should be treated as significantly lowered, in the 2nd percentile corridor [5–25 percentile] as lowered, in the 3rd and 4th [25–75 percentile] as medium, in the 5th [75–95 percentile] as increased and in the 6th [above the 95th percentile] as significantly increased. In order to form survey groups, it is necessary to use percentile limits of age-related electrical conductivity. The risk group should include the patients who have abnormally low values of age-related electrical conductivity of the breast, i.e. below the fifth percentile, which is the signal of high density of the acinar-ductal component of the breast for this age range. High density of acinar-ductal component is potentially dangerous since it may be combined with insufficient trophic function of connective tissue. It is a known fact that the ground substance of connective tissue plays the main role in the fulfillment of this function. Homeostasis disruption may lead to dystrophic processes including those in the basement membrane. Therefore, this method allows to detect the risk of tumorigenesis in women before the disease manifests itself, and it allows us to form risk groups for monitoring and correction of breast condition.

3. Early diagnostics of breast cancer

The electrical properties of cancer tumor differ greatly from the electrical properties of the surrounding tissues. It was established during several researches that malignant tumors have lower electrical impedance than normal tissues. The results of these studies are given in **Table 6** [29].

S. Haltiwanger published the results of several studies about the specific features of tumor cells that influence their electrical activity:

Authors, year	Frequency range investigated	Nature of study and results
Fricke et al. [29], 1926	20 kHz	They measured the parallel capacitance and resistance of the following excised samples from the breast—fat, gland, mastitis, fibroadenoma and carcinoma They found significantly higher permittivity of the tumor tissue at 20 kHz than the normal or benign tissues.
Singh et al. [30], 1979	100 Hz–100 kHz	They performed in vivo impedance measurements on female breasts with and without tumors. Their results showed that malignant tumors have higher relative permittivity and lower resistance than those of normal breast tissue
Chaudhary et al. [31], 1984	3 MHz–3 GHz	They examined excised normal and malignant breast tissues and found that the conductivity and permittivity of malignant tissues are higher than those of normal tissues, especially at frequencies lesser than 100 MHz.
Surowiec et al. [32], 1988	20 kHz–100 MHz	They conducted in vitro dielectric studies in three different samples of breast tissues—the main tumor tissue, the tissue immediately surrounding the tumor and the peripheral normal tissue. They found that the tumor tissues have a low-frequency (100 kHz) conductivity around 2–4 mS/cm which is higher than the conductivity of normal tissue (below 1 mS/cm) and lower than that of the tissue surrounding the tumor (8 mS/cm).
Morimoto et al. [33, 34], 1990	0–200 kHz	They measured the extracellular and intracellular resistances and membrane capacitance of breast tumors in vivo. They concluded that there are statistically significant differences between normal and cancerous tissues. However, it has been reported that malignant tumors have lowered capacitance compared to benign tumors. This is different from the results of the study conducted by Jossinet [36] and Fricke [33] which have recorded higher capacitance values for malignant tumors.
Jossinet [35], 1996	488 Hz–1 MHz	The study examined six groups of normal and pathological breast tissues in vitro. The variability of impedivity within each group was assessed by statistical methods. It was found that the variability was smaller in adipose tissue, carcinoma and fibroadenoma above 10 kHz.
Jossinet [36], 1998	488 Hz–1 MHz	Using the same data from [35], it was found that the cancerous tissue differed significantly from fibroadenoma and mammary gland tissues by the modulus of impedivity up to 31.25 kHz and from the remaining tissue groups (connective tissue, adipose tissue and mastopathy) by the low-frequency-limit resistivity and the phase angle from 125 kHz to 1 MHz. It was also observed that neither the impedivity nor the low-frequency-limit resistivity nor the fractional power value was different between the groups of normal and benign tissues.
Jossinet et al. [37], 1999	488 Hz–1 MHz	Again using the same excised data collected for previous studies, they defined a set of eight parameters that could differentiate cancerous breast tissues from noncancerous ones. They concluded that a combination of the parameters over various frequencies is necessary for the accurate differentiation among tissues.
Chauveau et al. [38], 1999	10 kHz–10 MHz	They conducted an in vitro study of normal and pathological breast tissues and observed significant differences in their dielectric properties. They have determined three indices based on extracellular resistance, intracellular resistance and membrane capacitance to differentiate between various tissue pathologies—normal, invasive ductal carcinoma (IDC), IDC with stromal reaction and fibrocystic changes.

Table 6.
The results of several researches of the electrical properties of cancer tumor.

1. Cancer cells have cell membranes that exhibit different electrochemical properties and a different distribution of electrical charges than normal tissues [30].

2. Cancer cells also have different lipid and sterol content than normal cells [31].

3. Cancer cells have altered membrane composition and membrane permeability, which results in the movement of potassium, magnesium and calcium out of the cell and the accumulation of sodium and water into the cell [32].

4. Cancer cells have lower potassium concentrations and higher sodium and water content than normal cells [33, 34].

5. The result of these mineral movements, membrane composition changes, energy abnormalities and membrane charge distribution abnormalities is a drop in the normal membrane potential and membrane capacitance.

6. An increase in the intracellular concentration of positively charged sodium ions and an increase in negative charges on the cell coat (glycocalyx) are two of the major factors causing cancerous cells to have lower membrane potential than healthy cells [31].

7. Two of the most outstanding electrical features of cancer cells are that they constantly maintain their membrane potential at a low value and their intracellular concentration of sodium at a high concentration [34, 35].

8. A sustained elevation of intracellular sodium may act as a mitotic trigger causing cells to go into cell division [35].

The results of the researches confirm that electrical conductivity is an appropriate parameter for the differentiation between healthy tissue and tumor tissue. The fundamental difference of electrical impedance scanning from other tomographic methods is that besides visual evaluation of the image, the electrical impedance mammography offers quantitative information [28]. If the diagnostic method under discussion yields a quantitative result, a value is defined, the overpassing of which is deemed to be a sufficient cause for qualitative evaluation, i.e. the so-called differentiation point. It is essential to define a precise differentiation point. The point with electrical conductivity exceeding 3 standard deviations [std] is considered to be the point of differentiation between breast cancer patients and healthy people. The detection of areas with high electrical conductivity exceeding 3 std. outside the lactiferous sinus in electrical impedance mammograms, which differs greatly from the electrical conductivity of normal breast tissue, is used as a diagnostic criteria for the detection of breast cancer [28]. Moreover, sizes of tumors as a rule do not exceed 10 mm.

Figure 3 shows the electrical impedance mammogram of a breast cancer patient with the following parameters: IC = 0.56, std. = 0.12. In the mammogram, at the 3 o'clock position near the areola, a focus without a sharp contour is visualized, its IC being equal to 0.94. Therefore, the IC in the area of interest exceeds the mammogram IC by more than 3 std.

Below X-ray images [fibroadipose involution, the upper external quadrant shows a mass less than 1 cm in size with uneven contour] and ultrasound mammograms [the external quadrant contains a lesion of irregular shape with uneven structure, 7 × 8 mm in size, with vascularization] of the same patient are presented.

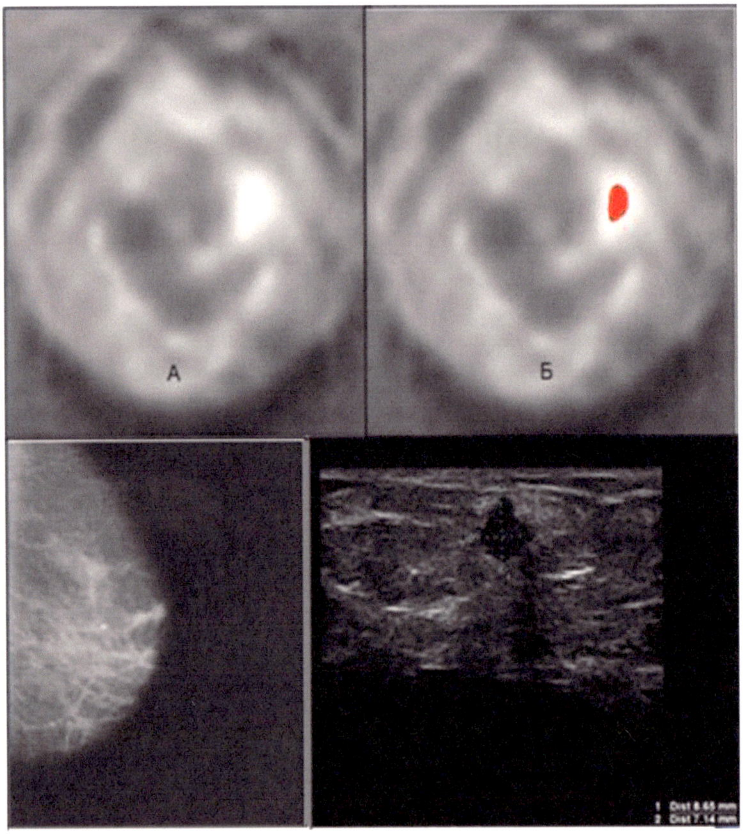

Figure 3.
Upper row: Electrical impedance mammogram of a breast cancer patient. At the 3 o'clock position near the areola a focus without a sharp contour, with abnormal electrical conductivity, is visualized. It is colored red (7 × 10 mm). The lower row shows X-ray and ultrasound images for the same patient.

For the last few years, clinical studies have been held in different countries determining the potential of electrical impedance mammography in breast cancer diagnostics. All these studies used electrical impedance computer mammograph MEIK v.5.6, abnormal electrical conductivity being the diagnostic criterion [28].

Sachin Prasad and colleagues performed a study to determine the diagnostic efficiency of 3D electrical impedance tomography [EIT] compared to mammography (mg) and ultrasonography (USG) in breast imaging [36]. A group of 88 patients with various breast complaints was examined using combined mammography and ultrasonography [MG & USG] or either of these modalities alone. The same patients were then examined using the 3D EIT imaging system MEIK. The study revealed that there was no overall significant difference in sensitivity between MG-USG [$p = 0.219$] and MG-EIT [$p = 0.779$] and USG-EIT [$p = 0.169$].

O. Raneta and colleagues [37] performed a study to analyze the possibilities of electrical impedance tomography [EIT] application in the differential diagnosis of pathologic lesions of the breast either solely or in combination with MMG/USG [37]. A group of 870 eligible women with suspected pathological breast lesion discovered by mammography [MMG] or ultrasound examination [USG] were recommended to pass histological examination to verify the diagnosis. The sensitivity of MMG increased from 87.8% when using it as an independent method to 94.5% with EIT added. The sensitivity of USG increased from 86.7% when used as an independent method to 93.3% with EIT added. The results of the study showed that the use of EIT in addition to MMG/USG can improve the sensitivity of these methods and increase the rate of early detection of breast cancer with minimal economic costs and time input of highly qualified staff.

Daglar and colleagues [38] performed a study to compare the usefulness of the breast electrical conductivity measures performed in a surgical examination room against conventional breast screening modalities for identifying the symptomatic lesions of the breast tissue [38]. A group of 181 patients were examined with ultrasonography [USG], mammography [MG] and electrical impedance scanning [EIS] modalities, which were followed up for 24 months to clarify the lesion tumor progression relationship. EIS exhibited compatible sensitivity [81.2%], accuracy [84.6%] and PPV [81.8%] rates with USG in BI-RADS 4 subgroup, combination of these modalities raised sensitivity rates to 92.31%, accuracy and PPV to 100%. EIS results in BI-RADS 3 subgroup were pointed out 77.8% specificity and 87.5% NPV rates. Breast electrical impedance measures should be useful to reduce the number of the unnecessary follow-up and biopsy rates in the clinical setting.

Xu Feng and colleagues [39] performed a study to investigate the diagnostic accuracy of electrical impedance tomography [EIT] for benign and malignant breast diseases in comparison to conventional ultrasonography and mammography [39]. A total of 121 patients with 126 breast lesions who underwent ultrasonography mammography and EIT were enrolled in the study. All of these lesions were confirmed by pathological biopsy. The accuracy, sensitivity, specificity, positive predictive value and negative predictive value of EIT, ultrasonography and mammography were calculated with histology used as the 'gold' standard. The accuracy of EIT, ultrasonography and mammography were 75.4, 81.7 and 76.1%, respectively. The sensitivity was 76.8, 94.6 and 74.4%, respectively. The specificity was 74.3, 71.4 and 77.6%, respectively. The accuracy, sensitivity and specificity of EIT combined with ultrasound in the diagnosis of breast lesions were 91.3, 98.2 and 85.7%, respectively. The accuracy [$\chi2 = 4.896$, $P = 0.027$] and specificity [$\chi2 = 4.242$, $P = 0.039$] were significantly higher on EIT than ultrasound. The accuracy, sensitivity and specificity of EIT combined with mammography were 95.5, 97.4 and 93.9%, respectively, which were significantly higher than those of mammography [$\chi2 = 13.474$, $P < 0.001$; $\chi2 = 8.573$, $P = 0.003$; $\chi2 = 5.333$, $P = 0.021$]. Used together with ultrasound or mammography, the electrical impedance tomography could be a valuable complementary examination in the diagnosis of breast diseases. Furthermore, EIT could provide very useful additional information for metabolic assessment of mammary glands, which may be used for early screening of breast diseases.

Blanca Murillo-Ortiz and colleagues [40] performed a study to know the effectiveness of the electrical impedance mammography for the detection of mammary carcinoma in 615 women from 25 to 70 years of age [40]. The sensitivity and specificity of the electrical impedance mammography (MEIK) was 85 and 97%, respectively.

Therefore, the studies showed high level of sensitivity and specificity, which allows to use abnormal electrical conductivity as the diagnostic criterion in screenings for early detection of breast cancer.

4. Distorted mammographic scheme in cases of breast cancer

Distortion of normal mammographic scheme appears in case of structural changes, such as pathological shadows and microcalcifications. These focal changes can be easily detected with the help of medical equipment checking the density of tissue. But along with focal changes, breast cancer can reveal itself through diffuse changes of breast structure, which also leads to the disruption of normal mammographic scheme, and this can be detected with electrical impedance mammography.

For X-ray diagnostics, diffuse changes are a difficult matter since they do not change the density of breast tissue.

As the disease develops, which leads to the destruction of the basement membrane of the epithelium, the lesion and surrounding tissues may undergo various phenomena followed by changes of electrical properties of the tumor mass:

- Edema and softening of fibrous connective tissue
- Slimming, hyalinosis, calcification
- Appearance of purulent areas
- Lymphocytic infiltration of tissue

Therefore, tumor growth is naturally accompanied by the changes of electrical properties of tumor and surrounding tissues. The criteria of distortion of normal mammographic scheme in cases of breast cancer are changes of contour, anatomical changes, local changes of electrical conductivity and change of comparative electrical conductivity. As previously stated, the electrical impedance method gives a possibility of quantitative imaging [28]. Quantitative analysis of an electrical impedance image allows to receive a histogram of electrical conductivity distribution and compares it with reference values. As a rule, distorted mammographic scheme in case of breast cancer is accompanied by changes of electrical conductivity of breast tissues. This phenomenon facilitates visual and quantitative interpretation of the lesion and can be used for diagnostic purposes. **Figure 4** shows several variants of distorted mammographic scheme in cases of breast cancer and their visual evaluation [1, contour deformation; 2,4, thickening of contour; 3, anatomic distortion; 5,6, local changes].

For the classification of a patient (healthy or affected), test of differences in the form of distributions [λ criterion], i.e. Kolmogorov-Smirnov test in Dx modification, is used [41]. This criterion, which is a nonparametric test, allows to determine the statistical value of differences in the distribution of any normal or abnormal features, including the distribution of electrical conductivity in electrical impedance tomograms. For the assessment of informativeness of distribution divergence, Kulback informativeness measure is applied [41]. High informativeness of the detected differences allows to refer the patient with high degree of probability to one class or the other (e.g. norm or cancer). In case of breast cancer, histogram of affected breast gets displaced, and Dx criterion exceeds 40% (**Figure 5**).

Table 7 shows the comparative electrical conductivity data for patients with breast cancer, benign changes, for healthy patients and for those with different types of breast structure; the data was received during clinical studies in the hospitals of Russia. It is evident that divergence of histograms of electrical conductivity distribution by more than 40% is observed only in cases of breast cancer, and actually divergence of histograms of electrical conductivity distribution by more than 30% in the majority of cases is observed during oncological processes in the breast.

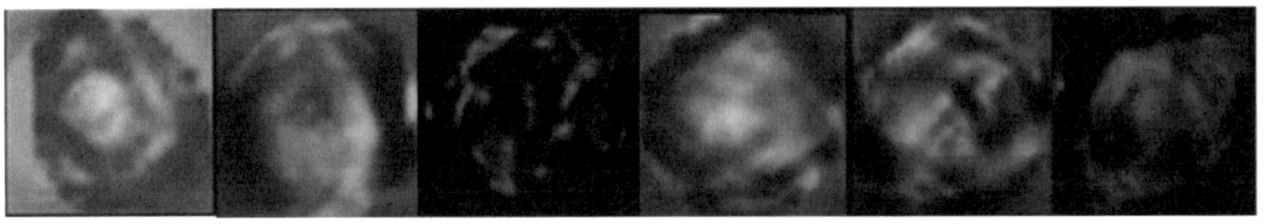

Figure 4.
Several variants of distorted mammographic scheme in cases of breast cancer.

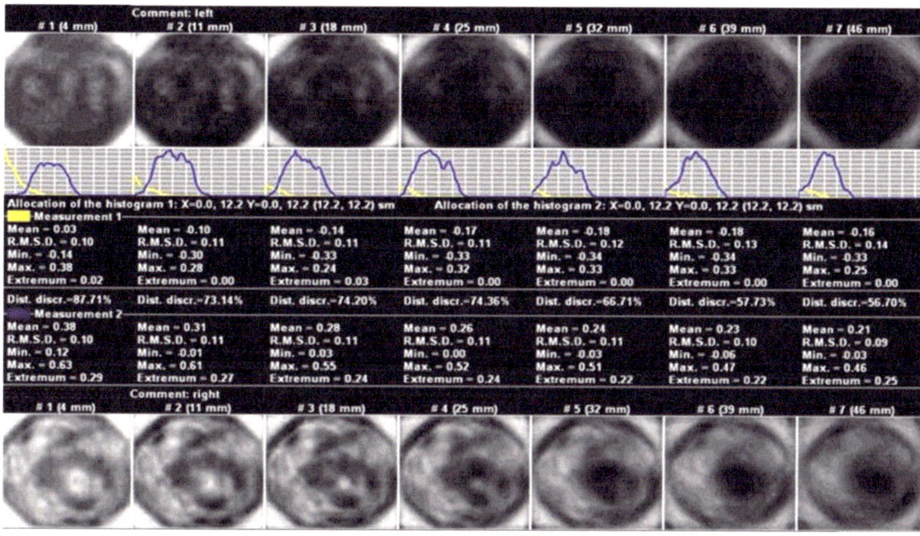

Figure 5.
Upper row, EIM. Seven scan planes. Breast cancer. Bottom row, EIM. Seven scan planes. Healthy breast. The second row shows the divergence between the histograms of electrical conductivity distribution of the affected and healthy breast.

	Number of patients	Comparative electric conductivity (affected – normal gland) <20%	20-30%	30-40%	40-50%	50-60%	>60%
Cancer	310	101 (33%)	67 (22%)	44 (14%)	37 (12%)	26 (8%)	35 (11%)
Healthy	161	157 (98%)	4 (2%)	0	0	0	0
Healthy acinar-ductal type	20	18 (90%)	1 (5%)	1 (5%)	0	0	0
Healthy amorphous type	32	28 (88%)	2 (6%)	2 (6%)	0	0	0
Benign	68	59 (87%)	7 (10%)	2 (3%)	0	0	0

Table 7.
Percentage distribution of healthy patients, patients with benign changes and breast cancer depending on the percentage of comparative electrical conductivity of the breasts.

EIM	ACR
Common scale	BI-RADS categories
No score	BI-RADS 0 poor image
0–1	BI-RADS 1 lesion is not defined
2–3	BI-RADS 2 benign tumors—routine mammography
4	BI-RADS 3 probably benign findings
5–7	BI-RADS 4 suspicious abnormality—biopsy
>8	BI-RADS 5 highly suggestive of malignancy—treatment/biopsy

Table 8.
EIM scale and ACR BI-RADS.

During the oncological process, natural changes of general and local electrical conductivity occur. And distortion of normal mammographic scheme may occur at an early stage of the disease. This is the reason why this criterion is included in the EIM scale of breast cancer diagnostics [41].

A scoring scale used for the evaluation of mass lesions in the breast by means of electrical impedance mammography allowed to relate the information received with BI-RADS ACR categorization (**Table 8**). The EIM scoring scale allowed to standardize the description of mass lesions examined by means of electrical impedance mammography and to use the patient follow-up algorithm developed by the American College of Radiology.

Therefore, the distortion of normal mammographic scheme along with abnormal electrical conductivity is one of the most frequent diagnostic indicators of breast cancer.

5. Discussion

Sensitivity and specificity are operational characteristics that allow to evaluate the effectiveness of a diagnostic method. Operational characteristics are influenced by several factors: size and area of pathology, age of patients in the groups under study and prevalence in the group under study. In the process of sensitivity and specificity calculation, the disease prevalence in the group is not taken into account. It is a significant benefit since it gives a possibility to spread the data received in a group of people onto other groups, with different prevalence. However, it is also a drawback of evaluation. The diagnostic test data should be spread cautiously onto groups of people that differ significantly from the group under study.

The calculation method used for operational characteristics such as sensitivity and specificity has its own peculiarities in cases of low and high prevalence.

Low-prevalence studies. As a rule, studies with low prevalence are preventive checkups. Screenings are low-prevalence studies as well.

Characteristics of screenings:

- Unrestricted population of sampling group, as a rule including many thousands of people
- Low prevalence
- Standard methodology
- Significant prevailing of healthy patients over patients with pathologies
- Impossibility to use reference method and histological verification of the diagnosis due to a large number of healthy patients
- Significant prevailing of patients with early stages of disease from among the number of those with revealed pathologies
- Impossibility to apply operational characteristics: specificity and sensitivity

High-prevalence studies. Studies performed in a diagnostic department of a specialized clinic are high-prevalence studies.

Characteristics of a diagnostic study:

- Restricted sampling population, several dozens of respondents

- High prevalence
- Standardized methodology
- Significant prevailing of patients with pathologies over healthy ones
- Significant prevailing of patients with progressing disease over those with early stages
- Use of referential method and histological verification of diagnosis
- Application of operational characteristics: sensitivity and specificity

Medium prevalence, which can be called an intermediate link, is a study held in a diagnostics department of a general practice clinic.

Characteristics of a diagnostic study:

- Unrestricted sampling population and timing
- Medium prevalence
- Standardized methodology
- Prevailing of healthy patients over patients with pathologies
- Full range of disease manifestation: from early-stage patients to patients with progressing disease
- Use of referential method and histological verification of diagnosis
- Application of operational characteristics: specificity and sensitivity

Is it correct to spread operational characteristics received from the second and third examples onto the screening?

1. Spreading the estimations received in high-prevalence conditions onto low-prevalence conditions should be done with caution. High-prevalence spectrum of disease manifestations differs from low-prevalence spectrum. Since diagnostic centers accumulate patients with a certain disease, in the structure of high-prevalence cases of progressing disease dominate significantly over early stages of disease.

2. Since every stage of disease has its own symptoms or specific criteria, for every stage the diagnostic criteria should have their own operational characteristics.

3. Operational characteristics are determined on the basis of restricted sample group of patients with verified diagnoses. Since reference tests, as a rule, are indifferent for the respondents, in such studies the number of persons not affected by the disease under study is minimal. In case of data spreading, it can influence the expected number of false-positive and false-negative results.

4. The optimal study for receiving operational characteristics of the method used from the point of view of patient selection, prevalence level, from the point of view of commonality of the methodology used and the usage of the reference

method and histological verification is not a low-prevalence study, such as screening, and is not a high-prevalence study as inpatient examination but a study held in an imaging room for the prevalence typical for the settlement. Shifting of operational characteristics in the situation of medium prevalence is preferable since it has a well-balanced data set.

Electrical impedance mammography is a tool for primary breast cancer screening. It is confirmed by its high informativeness, safety for the staff and patient, portability and mobility. Operational characteristics (sensitivity and specificity) are determined on a restricted sample group, the so-called high- and medium-prevalence group, with the use of reference method (X-ray mammography) and verified diagnosis. The studies were held in oncological centers and clinics. The study on a group of patients with high and medium prevalence demonstrated high sensitivity and specificity of the electrical impedance mammography. The received operational characteristics can be spread onto groups of patients with low prevalence and be used during planning of screening studies. It allows to use the electrical impedance mammography for primary breast cancer screening of big groups of population with low prevalence. The electrical impedance mammography fulfills its functional screening tasks without ionizing radiation and other potentially hazardous means. It can be used to perform examinations for women of all age groups in outpatient departments, schools, clinics for women, maternity hospitals and sanatoriums, i.e. in the gathering places for women. In such a way, the problem of organization of mass screening for women can easily be solved.

Conflict of interest

The authors declare no conflict of interest.

Author details

Alexander Karpov[1*], Marina Korotkova[2], Gregory Shiferson[3] and Elena Kotomina[4]

1 Department of Perinatal Diagnostics, Clinical Hospital #9, Yaroslavl, Russia

2 Head Women's Clinic, Clinical Hospital #9, Yaroslavl, Russia

3 Department of Obstetrics and Gynecology, Yaroslavl State Medical Academy, Russia

4 Department of Ultrasound Diagnostics, Yaroslavl Regional Oncology Hospital, Russia

*Address all correspondence to: Karpovay@medyar.ru

References

[1] Wilson JMG, Jungner G. Handbook Principles and Practice of Screening for Disease Dedicated to Screening of Diseases. World Health Organization; 1968

[2] Barchuk AA, Belyaev AM, Filochkina AV, Arseniev AI. Cancer screening and mortality. Anssi Auvinen практическая онкология, Т. 2016;**17**(4)

[3] Gabriel, Domchek. Breast cancer in young women. Breast Cancer Research. 2010;**12**:212

[4] Berrington De González A, Reeves G. Mammographic screening before age 50 years in the UK: Comparison of the radiation risks with the mortality benefits. British Journal of Cancer. 2005;**93**(5, 5):590-596

[5] Breast Screening Programme, England. Statistics for 2004-15. Health & Social Care Information Centre. Published 24 February 2016

[6] Britton P, Warwick J, Wallis MG, O'keeffe S, Taylor K, Sinnatamby R, et al. Measuring the accuracy of diagnostic imaging in symptomatic breast patients: Team and individual performance. The British Journal of Radiology. 2012;**85**:415-422

[7] Leung et al. Can breast magnetic resonance imaging demonstrate characteristic finding of preoperative ductal carcinoma in situ in Taiwanese woman? Asian Journal of Surgery. 2010;**33**(3):143-149

[8] Nagao Y, Kawaguchi Y, Sugiyama Y, Saji S, Kashiki Y. Relationship between mammographic density and the risk of breast cancer in Japanese women: A case-control study. Breast Cancer. 2003;**10**(3):228-233

[9] Boyd et al. Mammographic densities and breast cancer risk. Cancer Epidemiology, Biomarkers & Prevention. 1998;**7**:1133-1144

[10] Kolb et al. Comparison of the performance of screening mammography, physical examination, and breast US and evaluation of factors that influence them: An analysis of 27,825 patient evaluations. Radiology. 2002;**225**(1):165-175

[11] McCormack, Santos, et al. Breast density and parenchymal pattern as markers of breast cancer risk: A meta-analysis. Cancer Epidemiology, Biomarcers & Prevention. 2006;**15**(6):1159-1169

[12] Leung et al. Will screening mammography in the east do more harm than good? American Journal of Public Health. 2002;**92**(11):1841-1846

[13] Hammerstein et al. Absorbed radiation dose in mammography. Radiology. 1979;**130**:485-491

[14] Brenner DJ, Sawant SG, Hande MP, et al. Routine screening mammography: How important is the radiation-risk side of the benefit-risk equation? International Journal of Radiation Biology. 2002;**78**:1065-1067

[15] Heyes GJ, Mill AJ, Charles MW. Enhanced biological effectiveness of low energy X-rays and implications for the UK breast screening programme. The British Journal of Radiology. 2006;**79**:195-200

[16] Hoekstra P. Quantitative digital thermology: 21st century imaging systems. In: Paper Presented at: OAND Conference, Hamilton, Ontario. 2001

[17] Son et al. Changing patterns in the clinical characteristics of Korean patients with breast cancer during the last 15 years. Archives of Surgery. 2006;**141**(2):155-160

[18] Breast Cancer Risk Factors: A Review of the Evidence. Surry Hills, NSW: National Breast and Ovarian Cancer Centre; 2009

[19] Destounis S, Arieno A, Morgan R, Roberts C, Chan A. Qualitative versus quantitative mammographic breast density assessment: Applications for the US and Abroad. MDPI Diagnostics. 2017

[20] Boyd NF, Byng JW, Jong RA, Fishell EK, Little LE, Miller AB, et al. Quantitative classification of mammographic densities and breast cancer risk: Results from the Canadian National Breast Screening Study. Journal of the National Cancer Institute. 1995;**87**(9):670-675

[21] Pike MC, Pearce CL, Wu AH. Prevention of cancers of the breast, endometrium and ovary. Oncogene. 2004;**23**:6379-6391 USC/Norris Cancer Center, Los Angeles, CA, USA

[22] Kelemen LE, Pankratz VS, Sellers TA, Brandt KR, Wang A, Janney C, et al. Age-specific trends in mammographic density: The Minnesota breast Cancer family study. American Journal of Epidemiology. 2008;**167**:1027-1036

[23] Greendale GA, Reboussin BA, Slone S, Wasilauskas C, Pike MC, Ursin G. Postmenopausal hormone therapy and change in mammographic density. Journal of the National Cancer Institute. 2003;**95**:30-37

[24] Maskarinec G, Pagano I, Lurie G, Kolonel LN. A longitudinal investigation of mammographic density: The multiethnic cohort. Cancer Epidemiology, Biomarkers & Prevention. 2006;**15**:732-739

[25] McTiernan A, Martin CF, Peck JD, Aragaki AK, Chlebowski RT, Pisano ED, et al. Estrogen-plus-progestin use and mammographic density in postmenopausal women: Women's Health initiative randomized trial. Journal of the National Cancer Institute. 2005;**97**:1366-1376

[26] McCormack VA, dos Santos Silva I. Breast density and parenchymal patterns as markers of breast cancer risk: A meta-analysis. Cancer Epidemiology, Biomarkers & Prevention. 2006;**15**(6):1159-1169

[27] Supplemental Screening for Breast Cancer in Women with Dense Breasts: A Systematic Review for the U.S. Preventive Service Task Force. Agency for Healthcare Research and Quality, U.S. Department of Health and Human Services; 2016

[28] Karpov A et al. Diagnostic system in electrical impedance mammography. Background. In: Malik AM, editor. Handbook "New Perspectives in Breast Imaging". 2018

[29] Ng EYK, Vinitha Sree S, Ng KH, Kaw G. The use of tissue electrical characteristics for breast cancer detection: A perspective review. Technology in Cancer Research and Treatment. August 2008;**7**(4):1533-0346

[30] Cure JC. On the electrical characteristics of cancer. In: Paper Presented at the Second International Congress of Electrochemical Treatment of Cancer, Florida. 1995

[31] Revici E. Research in Pathophysiology as Basis for Guided Chemotherapy, with Special Application to Cancer. Princeton, NJ: D. Van Nostrand Company; 1961

[32] Seeger PG, Wolz S. Successful Biological Control of Cancer: By Combat against the Causes. Gesamtherstellung: Neuwieder Verlagsgesellschaft mbH; 1990

[33] Cone CD. The role of surface electrical transmembrane potential in normal and malignant mitogenesis. Annals of the New York Academy of Sciences. 1975;**238**:420-435

[34] Cope FW. A medical application of the Ling Association-induction hypothesis: The high potassium, low sodium diet of the Gerson cancer therapy. Physiological Chemistry and Physics. 1978;**10**(5):465-468

[35] Cone CD. Transmembrane Potentials and Characteristics of Immune and Tumor Cells. Boca Raton, FL: CRC Press; 1985

[36] Sachin Prasad N, Houserkova D, Campbell J. Breast imaging using 3D electrical impedence tomography. Biomedical Papers of the Medical Faculty of the University Palacky, Olomouc, Czech Republic. 2008;**152**(1):151-154

[37] Raneta O, Bella V, Bellova L, Zamecnikova E. The use of electrical impedance tomography to the differential diagnosis of pathological mammographic/sonographic findings. Neoplasma. 2013;**60**(6):647-654

[38] Daglar G, Senol K, Yakut ZI, Yuksek YN, Tutuncu T, Tez M, et al. Effectiveness of breast electrical impedance imaging for clinically suspicious breast lesions. Bratislava Medical Journal. 2016;**117**(9):505-510

[39] Feng X, Mengxin L, Peter J, Hongchuan J. Utilisation of electrical impedance tomography and/or ultrasound and mammography in breast disease diagnosis: A controlled study. National Medical Journal of China. 2017;**97**(18):1391-1395

[40] Murillo-Ortiz B, et al. Diagnosis of breast cancer by electrical impedance mammography MEIK. Revista Mexicana de Mastología. 2019;**9**:20-27

[41] Karpov A et al. Electrical impedance mammographic scheme norm and pathology. In: Handbook « Mammoraphy. Techniques and Review». 2015

Chapter 2

Detection of Breast Cancer in Mammograms through a New Features Technique

Anwar Yahy Ebrahim

Abstract

This research proposes a new framework for detection of breast cancer in mammograms. It extracts certain dynamic features to distinguish between benign and malignant mammograms. To this aim, this framework uses set of various techniques. First step we have achieved improvement on breast mammogram to improve the image accuracy based on this framework, after new method has been used for features extraction. New methods named Sparse Principal Component Analysis and Weighted Sparse Principal Component Analysis are used to select the distinctive features of the mammograms. The analyzed mammograms are then identified as benign or malignant through codebook technique is more efficient than other on the MIAS data set. The proposed framework tested on MIAS data set achieved an overall classification accuracy of 98% with codebook classifier for sequential selection of benign and malignant mammograms. Suggested method achieves good results when we have verified on various mammograms.

Keywords: chest cancer, mammograms feature extraction, weighted features, codebook design technique

1. Introduction

There are a number of renowned and probable causes for chest cancer. These can be split into seven broad classes: hormonal factors, age, proliferate chest disease, family history of chest cancer, lifestyle factors and [1–5]. Estimates show with the development of technology, radiation scientists have the opportunity to advance their interpretation of image using computer technology capabilities that can develop image resolution from mammography [6–11]. A variety of computer assisted diagnostic systems were proposed such as [12, 13]. In this paper, enhanced Principle Component Analysis (PCA) was used to extract features. Although PCA has been widely applied in the area, but the features considered in this study have not been extracted before [14]. Further, these extracted features are reduced to the best features only. This process is accomplished by two variations of PCA as Sparse Principle Component Analysis (SPCA) [15, 16] and Weighted Sparse Principle Component Analysis (WSPCA). The choice of the (ideally "small") number of principal components (PCs)to include into the description of the data without losing too much information was somewhat arbitrary [14]. Codebooks represents is final optimized codebook for samples will be generated. It can represent the attributes of the mammograms images more adequately. Proposed technique realized quite perfect. Project is ordered displayed in stage first. Stage second presents related work. Stage third defines the suggested method. Stage forth contains experimental outcomes and conclusion is presented in stage fifth.

2. Proposed technique

The projected method is split into four major phases as presented in **Figure 1**. The first phase is representing enhancement by applying histogram equalization, the second phase is representing feature selection, the third phase is representing codebook and the final phase is representing Design Classifier. Every part of these four phases is defined below one after another.

2.1 Enhancement for image

In this phase, the improvement is focused in flat regions avoid over development decreased influence of edge shadowing.

2.2 Features extraction

Features play an important applied DCT projected method.

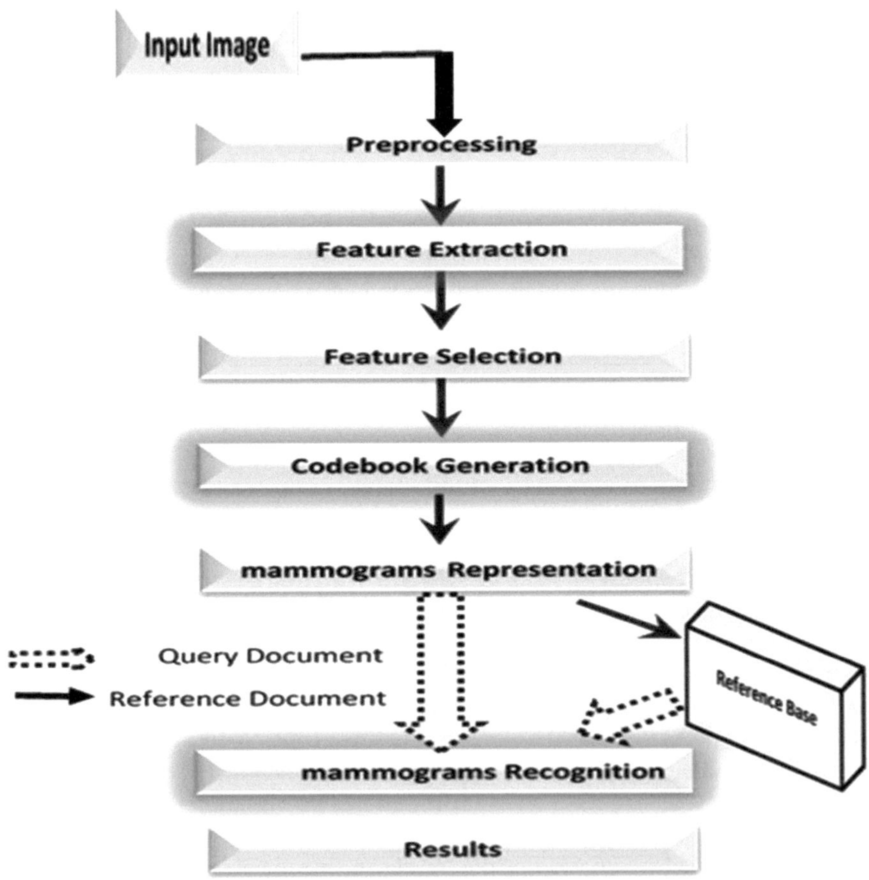

Figure 1.
Projected technique.

2.2.1 Discrete cosine transform (DCT)

Features Discrete cosine transform (DCT) is applied for converting the signal into its frequency parts. DCT has the property of separability and symmetry. 2-Dimensional DCT of the input is presented by the following equation:

$$\mathrm{C}\ (\mathrm{u},\mathrm{v}) = a(u)a(v)\sum_{x=0}^{N-1}\sum_{y=0}^{N-1} f(x,y)\cos\left[\frac{\pi(2x+1)u}{2N}\right]\cos\left[\frac{\pi(2y+1)V}{2N}\right] \quad (1)$$

where $0 \le \mathrm{u} \le \mathrm{N}$, & $0 \le \mathrm{v} \le \mathrm{N}$, and $a(u)a(v) = \begin{cases} \sqrt{\frac{1}{N}} & for v, u \neq 0 \\ \sqrt{\frac{2}{N}} & for u, v = 0 \end{cases}$

2.3 Feature selection

In the past, researchers used to reduce the dimensions apply PCA here. Each PC is basically a linear combination of all the original features. This makes the results difficult to interpret [14, 16]. Various approaches have been attempted to overcome this problem. We present a novel technique called WSPCA applying LASSO (elastic net) to generate modified PCs with sparse loadings. Important features are selected based on their weights. The aim behind is to use WSPCA to construct a regression framework in which PCA is reconstructed exactly, and use LASSO to construct modified PCs with sparse loadings. Then important features are selected with adaptive feature's weights to find the best loading vector corresponding the features to achieve high accuracy. The uncorrelated linear combinations are called principal components, which express maximal variations in the data. This provided the researchers with a method of transforming the original high-dimensional dataset into one of the much lower dimension. This method was devised inevitably at the cost of some information loss (variance) and limited ability to interpret new variables and analysis. SPCA can successfully derive sparse loadings.

Despite of its positive aspects, SPCA is not efficient in identifying important features with high accuracy. It also lacks a better step to choose its regulation parameter [14, 16]. WSPCA uses strict criterion and flexible control for selected the important features. To fit our WSPCA models for both features weights expression arrays and regular multivariate features, an efficient algorithm is proposed. In addition, we propose a novel form to calculate the total difference of the modified PCs. In this study, the algorithm for WSPACA in parallel to PCA and SPCA is presented in detail with example: let DCT features (variables) F = (F1, F2... Fp)' represent a p-dimensional random vector with a multivariate normal distribution. It is possible that some features correlate with one another. For instance, if the variables F1 and F2 are highly correlated, such that the correlation index between F1 and F2 approaches 0.9, then either F1 or F2 could be eliminated from the analysis as its role is duplicated by the other. By doing this, the basis of the original features is altered to a more efficient set by using linear combinations. In the general p-dimensional case, this leads to a candidate set of new features. The explained steps are presented in Algorithm 1.

Algorithm 1

Step 1: Suppose A beginning at V [1: k], the loadings of the headmost k (PCs).

Step 2: Assumed a constant A = $[\alpha_1 ... \alpha_k]$, fix the next elastic net issue

$$X_W = \sum_{j=1}^{n} W_j X_j \text{ , j = 1, ...,n} \quad (2)$$

Step 3: $\beta_{WSPCAj} = \left(\left|\alpha_j^T X_W{}^T X_W\right| - \frac{\lambda_{1,j}}{2}\right) + Sign\left(\alpha_j^T X_W{}^T X_W\right)$, j = 1,..,k (3)

Step 4: For a fixed β_j = [βSPCA1,...,βSPCkf], PCA can be found via compute the SVD of the features matrix, calculate the SVD of XWTXW = UDVT, (4)

then update A = UVT. (5)

Step 5: reiterate Steps 4–5, until concourse.

Step 6: Normalization : $\hat{V}_j = \frac{\beta_{WSPCA_j}}{\|\beta_{WSPCA_j}\|}$ (6)

In step 1, the presented PCs are the linear combinations of all original features, V is the response vector (nonzero components) and it is less than or equal to k, given an integer k with $1 \le k \le p$. In Step 2, A is a vector matrix. In Step 3, assumed variables of X are presented in $(n \times p)$ matrix, where n rows represent an independent feature from features (number of observations) and p is the number of variables (dimensions), where is spare coefficients, j be the predictors for nonzero entries, is feature vector, XTX is represent (covariance matrix) transpose for vector matrix by row vector of features, where represents the norm in the constraint. In the present research, in order to find the optimal number of features, λ is penalty by directly imposing a constraint on PCA and λ1, j = 0 call SPCA criterion r. B = (β0, β1, β2,., βk)T, where its regression coefficients represent the optimal minimizing. In Step 4, SVD is a singular value decomposition, UD are PCs, the columns of V^T are the consistent loading of the PCs eigenvectors, V diagonalizes the covariance matrix XTX, U are called Eigen values of the covariance matrix, D is the diagonal matrix, which has the eigenvalues of covariance matrix. XTX and V are the Eigen—genes, which represent the sparse loading of feature matrix. In Step 6, W_j is weighted features, and, βj = [βSPCA1,..., βSPCAf]. Then (XW) was calculated, which represents weighted feature matrix. Where X is a new feature matrix of SPCA and represents eight types of features.

Coefficients for WSPCA technique were obtained by minimizing both SPCA and weighted feature matrix [17, 18]. In Step 7, represents highly correlated by weighted features among all features, is penalty by directly imposing an constraint on PCA and (λ1, j = 0), represents to exclude redundant features with very little variation from other features that sufficiently represents it. This is where adaptive weights were used for penalizing different coefficients in the 1 penalty, Here, we can ignore the penalty part in calculating Step 8.

Then, AW = UVT was updated where PCs were selected for displaying the selected features. Thus, a large dimensionality decrease was realized. Then after (Vj), normalization was calculated for approximated weighted sparse principal components. Step 9 was where βWSPCA was the WSPCA coefficient.

2.4 Codebook design

After representing each set of features, hierarchical clustering groups the features selection based on similarity to build a hierarchy of clusters. This clustering approach starts with each object as a single class and merges objects into the classes until all objects are in one cluster [18, 19]. The proposed technique needs to define a dimension measure allowing comparison of two classes. The operation of a hierarchical clustering is illustrated in **Figure 2**.

As an example, seven labeled patterns are shown in **Figure 2a**, in this research these seven labeled pattern can be consider as seven fragmented windows, which is

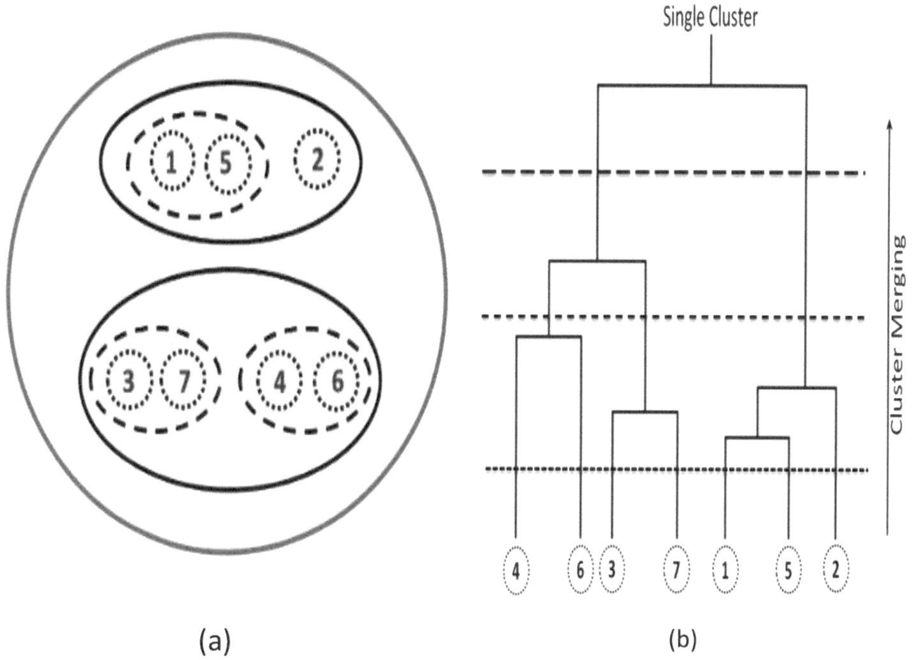

Figure 2.
Points falling in hierarchical cluster in (a) and binary tree of hierarchical clustering in (b).

then group together in a single cluster. **Figure 2b** represents the binary tree corresponding to the patterns in **Figure 2a**. In the binary tree, each patterns are the leaves, each branching points are the similarity between sub-trees. Horizontal cuts using different line patterns in the tree represents classes.

The distance between the two classes can be calculated as the minimum, maximum or the average of the dimensions between attributes of patterns in different clusters. This research employed the average-link method for clustering. In this method, the distance between two categories is defined as the average of the dimensions between all the objects in the two categories. This method is expressed by the next equation.

$$Dist(c_i, c_j) = \underset{x \in c_i, y \in c_j}{avg} Dist(x, y) \tag{7}$$

where, c_i and c_j be two categories. Dist defines the dimension between c_i and c_j.

In addition, since the number of classes for each mammogram is not known, this study uses the distance criterion to represent the number of cluster. For each mammogram the proposed technique generates the clusters from the important features. In this research, the important features clusters are also termed as codebooks.

3. Outcomes and discussion

We have applied widely presented datasets MIAS [20]. The database image of 69 mammograms were being benign, 54 malignant also 207 normal Improvement has been done by histogram equalization. Outcomes have been display in **Figure 3**. Once the codebook for important features are generated, the proposed technique sorts the classes according to the cardinality and keeps only those classes which have sufficient number of features. As a codebook produced from feature selection are illustrated in **Figure 3**, respectively.

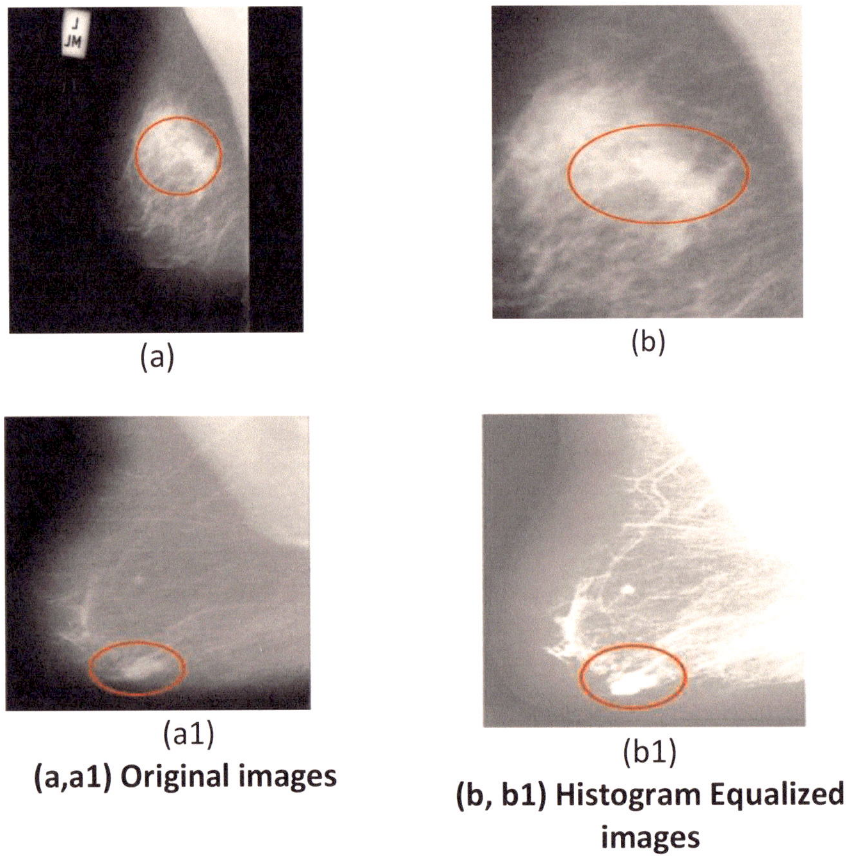

Figure 3.
Results by histogram equalization (a, a1); original images (b, b1); and histogram equalized images.

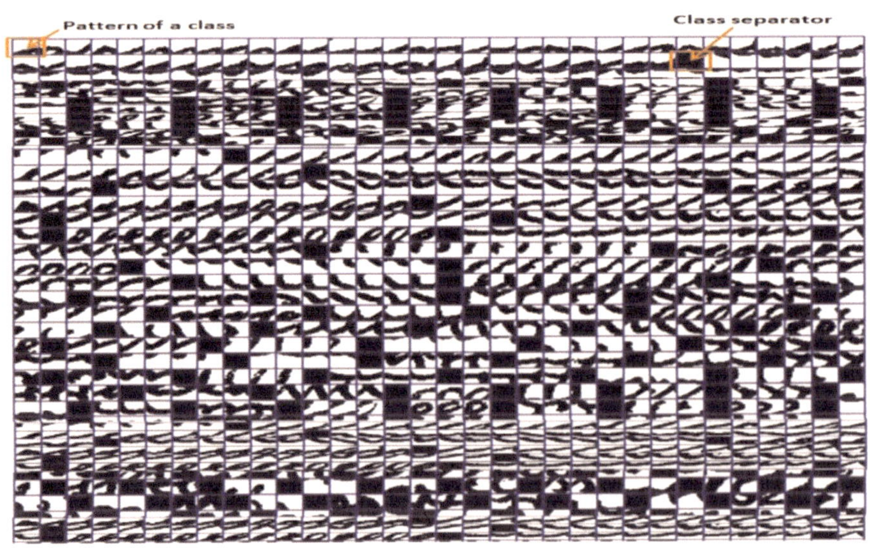

Figure 4.
Mammograms: codebook obtained from the important features on a mammograms sample.

In codebook there are different number classes. Each class contains relatively homogeneous groups of similar forms, which are dissimilar to elements in the other classes. These classes are separated by the black window in the codebook as illustrated in **Figure 4**.

Once the codebook is generated for each mammograms sample, the next step is to determine how to use this information to represent mammograms sample recognition as discussed in the following section.

4. Verification

These codebooks contain different information about a mammograms image and complement each other. It would therefore be a good idea the codebooks to compare two mammogram images. When two mammogram images are compared, the proposed technique computes the distance between them using their codebooks. The final dimension between the two mammogram samples is calculated as a weighted combination of the two distances (**Table 1**).

Techniques	SPCA technique (%)	WSPCA technique (%)
SVM	88	89
Bayesian	89	91
Decision tree	94	95
Codebook design	96	98

Table 1.
Comparison of achievement measurement of various classifiers with SPCA and WSPCA techniques.

5. Conclusion

Suggested method is improved for test the breast cancer from mammograms. This technique achieves this testing in multiple stages. The preprocessing stage on improve image accuracy. Features selection by SPCA and WSPCA has been achieved. Codebook generated for each mammograms sample represent classify as a normal or nonnormal. The tests display projected method provides especially perfect outcomes.

Author details

Anwar Yahy Ebrahim
Department of Computer Science, Babylon University, Babylon, Iraq

*Address all correspondence to: anwaralawady@gmail.com

References

[1] Naveed N, Choi TS, Jaffar MA. Malignancy and abnormality detection of mammograms using DWT features and ensembling of classifiers. International Journal of the Physical Sciences. 2011;**6**(8):2107-2116

[2] Wallis M, Walsh M, Lee J. A review of false negative mammography in a symptomatic population. Clinical Radiology. 1991;**44**:13-15

[3] Tang J, Rangayyan R, Xu J, El Naqa I, Yang Y. Computer-aided detection and diagnosis of breast cancer with mammography: Recent advances. IEEE Transactions on Information Technology in Biomedicine. 2009;**13**(2): 236-251

[4] Kom G, Tiedeu A, Kom M. Automated detection of masses in mammograms by local adaptive thresholding. Computers in Biology and Medicine. 2007;**37**(1):37-48

[5] Eltonsy N, Tourassi G, Elmaghraby A. A concentric morphology model for the detection of masses in mammography. IEEE Transactions on Medical Imaging. 2007; **26**(6):880-889

[6] Wang X, Zheng B, Good WF, King JL, Chang Y. Computer assisted diagnosis of breast cancer using a data-driven bayesian belief network. International Journal of Medical Informatics. 1999;**54**(2):115-126. Techniques Accuracy (%) Sensitivity (%) Specificity (%) KNN 76.2 77.2 77.5 Neural Network 85.3 84.1 85.3 SVM 86.3 87 87.3 Bayesian 87.3 89.3 89.6 International Journal of Multimedia and Ubiquitous Engineering. 2012;7(2):363

[7] Kaul K, Daguilh FM-L. Early detection of breast cancer, is mammography enough. Hospital Physician. 2002;**38**(9):49-54

[8] Brodersen J, Siersma VD. Long-term psychosocial consequences of false-positive screening mammography. The Annals of Family Medicine. 2013;**11**(2): 106-115

[9] Kendall EJ, Flynn MT. Automated breast image classification using features from its discrete cosine transform. PLoS One. 2014;**9**(3):e91015

[10] Mavroforakis M, Georgiou H, Dimitropoulos N, Cavouras D, Theodoridis S. Significance analysis of qualitative mammographic features, using linear classifiers, neural networks and support vector machines. European Journal of Radiology. 2004;**54**(1):80-89

[11] Daskalakis A, et al. An efficient CLAHE-based, spot adaptive, image segmentation technique for improving microarray genes' quantification. In: 2nd International Conference on Experiments/Process/System Modelling/Simulation and Optimization; Athens; 2007

[12] Strang G. The discrete cosine transform. SIAM Review. 1999;**41**(1): 135-147

[13] Duda R, Hart PE, Stork DG. Pattern Classification. 2nd ed. New York: John Wiley and Sons; 2001

[14] Jolliffe IT, Trendafilov NT, Uddin M. A modified principal component technique based on the LASSO. Journal of Computational and Graphical Statistics. 2003;**12**(3):531-547

[15] Jolliffe IT. Principal Component Analysis. 1st ed. Springer-Verlag; 1986. p. 487

[16] Hui ZOU, Hastie T, Tibshirani R. Sparse principal component analysis. Journal of Computational and Graphical

Statistics. 2006;**15**(2):265-286. DOI: 10.1198/106186006X113430,2006

[17] Ebrahim AY. Detection of breast cancer in mammograms through a new features and decision tree based, classification framework. Journal of Theoretical and Applied Information Technology. 2017;**95**(12):6256-6267. ISSN: 1992–8645

[18] Ebrahim AY, Sulong G. Offline handwritten signature verification using back propagation artificial neural network matching technique. Journal of Theoretical and Applied Information Technology. 2014;**65**(3):790-800

[19] Ebrahim AY. Classification of Arabic autograph as genuine and forged through a combination of new attribute extraction techniques. Journal of University of Babylon. 2017;**25**(5): 1873-1885

[20] Suckling J et al. The mammographic image analysis society digital mammogram database Exerpta Medica. International Congress Series. 1994; **1069**:375-378

Chapter 3

Breast Cancer and *BRCA1* and *BRCA2* Pathogenic Variants

Naren Basu and D. Gareth Evans

Abstract

Breast cancer remains the most common female cancer worldwide. The majority will arise spontaneously, with almost a third having a heritable component. Approximately 5–10% of all breast cancers will have a strong inherited element with pathogenic variants in the *BRCA1* and *BRCA2* amongst the most studied breast cancer genes. An overview of breast cancer is provided with references to the clinical and pathological features in *BRCA1* and *BRCA2* related cancers. The roles of PARP inhibitors and immunotherapy are discussed. The management of healthy individuals harbouring a pathogenic variant in the two genes is reviewed and future directions considered.

Keywords: *BRCA1*, *BRCA2*, breast cancer, risk reduction, mastectomy, pathogenic variant

1. Introduction

Breast cancer remains the most common cancer amongst women in the world [1]. In the UK, 25% of all female cancers originate from the breast with estimates that 1 in 7–10 will develop this disease during their lifetime [2]. In 2018, there were over 2 million new cases of breast cancer worldwide, accounting for almost 12% of all cancer [3]. In developed countries, almost 80% of breast cancers occur in post-menopausal women, predominantly in the Caucasian population.

Breast cancer represents a heterogenous disease process and an understanding of the clinical aspects is required prior to appreciating the aspects of breast cancer amongst *BRCA1/2* pathogenic variant (PV) carriers.

2. Invasive or *in-situ* (non-invasive cancer)

The vast majority of breast cancers are invasive (up to 90%) presenting via a symptomatic pathway. In contrast, *in-situ* disease tends to be more commonly identified via breast screening programmes (e.g., NHSBSP) with advances in digital mammography or incidentally. In the USA, *in situ* disease comprises almost 25% of all breast cancers, 80% of which are identified by breast screening [4].

In histopathological terms, invasive cancers will have breached the basement membrane with metastatic potential compared with the more innocuous *in-situ* disease where the disease process is contained within the basement membrane, with theoretically limited or no metastatic potential.

IntechOpen

3. Ductal or lobular origin

The microanatomy of the breast can be considered to comprise of terminal ductal lobular unit [5, 6]. Each breast lobule is by a collecting duct terminating in the lobule. This serves as the basic functional unit of the breast. Invasive ductal carcinoma (also termed no special type carcinoma) represents the most common type of breast cancer accounting for almost 80% of cancer. Invasive lobular carcinoma is less common accounting for almost 10% of cases.

These two types of breast cancer are biologically different. Invasive lobular cancers tend to have a more spreading growth pattern, meaning that they can be more difficult to diagnose or size on routine mammograms or clinical examination. In addition, they may be resistant to neo-adjuvant chemotherapy. Invasive lobular cancers tend to be more hormone-sensitive, HER2 negative and lower grade breast cancer (see below).

4. Grade of breast cancer

This refers to the microscope assessment of the breast cancer and determining how the cells look compared with normal breast tissue [6]. This in turn will predict the biological activity of the breast cancer, with high-grade tumours considered to be faster growing with a more aggressive behaviour.

4.1 Grades in in-situ disease

Low grade—slow growing and more closely resemble normal breast tissue.

Moderate/intermediate grade—more abnormal looking compared with low grade, with a more rapid growth pattern.

High grade—cells look quite different to normal breast tissue, grow quicker with an increased chance of progressing to an invasive cancer.

4.2 Grades in invasive cancer

There are three different grades of invasive breast cancer based on an assessment of tubule formation, nuclear pleomorphism and mitotic count:

Grade 1 (well differentiated).

Grade 2 (moderately differentiated).

Grade 3 (poorly differentiated).

5. Hormone receptor status

Oestrogen receptors (ER) were first identified in 1958 (Elwood, Chicago) but an appreciation of the hormonal component of breast cancer predates this to the 1890s when George Beatson performed oophorectomy as a treatment for breast cancer in women [7]. It still remains a critical biological factor in the modern day management of breast cancer.

The oestrogen (ER) and progesterone receptors (PR) relevant to breast cancer are intracellular receptors that are activated by the hormone oestrogen (17 beta oestrodiol) acting as a DNA-binding transcription factor, in particular stimulation of mammary cells.

Approximately 70–80% of breast cancers overexpress ER [8]. These hormone sensitive breast cancers may be treated with anti-hormone therapy by either selective oestrogen receptor modulators (e.g., Tamoxifen) or aromatase inhibitors.

6. HER2 receptor status

The HER2 receptor (human epidermal growth factor receptor) is a transmembrane tyrosine kinase that is overexpressed in 15–20% of breast cancers [9]. Amplification of this oncogene is considered a marker of aggressiveness and is an important biomarker for targeted therapy. Drugs targeting the HER2 receptor (e.g., Trastuzumab, Pertuzumab) have significantly altered the clinical outcomes of otherwise poor prognosis HER2 positive breast cancers.

7. Molecular subtypes of breast cancer

Gene expression profiling has enabled molecular classification of breast cancer into intrinsic subtypes [10] that include:

1. Luminal A: hormone receptor positive (ER/PR +ve) and HER2 negative. They express low levels of the protein Ki-67, a cellular marker for proliferation. These cancers tend to be low grade, slow growing, good prognosis cancers.

2. Luminal B: hormone receptor positive (ER/PR +ve) and either HER2 positive or negative with a high level of Ki-67 expression. Faster growing and worse prognosis than luminal A cancers.

3. Triple negative breast cancer (TNBC)/basal-like: these are hormone receptor negative and HER2 negative (ER/PR/HER2 −ve). This accounts for 10–20% of all breast cancers, more commonly found in women with a *BRCA1* PV, young women and African-American women. It is a rapidly growing, poor prognosis cancer.

4. HER2-enriched: these are HER2 positive and ER/PR negative cancer (HER2 +ve, ER/PR −ve). They tend to grow faster than luminal cancers but can be treated with targeted therapies.

8. Treatments for breast cancer

The management of breast cancer is a multi-modal delivered in a multidisciplinary setting. In brief, treatments include:

8.1 Surgery

Excision of the breast lesion and assessment of the axillary lymph node for regional metastasis. Historically this involved mastectomy with axillary clearance, which has now been refined following some seminal trial in breast cancer surgery to offering appropriate women breast conserving surgery ("lumpectomy") and sentinel node biopsy. There are still important indications for mastectomy that would include genetic mutation status, family history, previously treated breast cancer, inflammatory breast cancer and patient choice.

8.2 Anti endocrine therapy

Hormone sensitive breast cancers are treated with anti hormonal therapy for a minimum period of 5 years that can be extended to 10–15 years based on recent emerging data. There is an improved overall survival, reduced recurrence rate and reduction in the incidence of a contralateral breast cancer.

8.3 Radiotherapy

This is a localised, targeted therapy of high-energy X-rays that complements breast conservation surgery in almost all cases of invasive cancer, reducing local recurrence rates by almost 20–30% [11]. It may be offered following mastectomy if there is a high burden of disease.

8.4 Chemotherapy

This systemic treatment may be offered pre surgery (neo adjuvant) or post surgery (adjuvant). The choice of chemotherapy regimen is determined by number factors and may include anthracycline-taxane combinations. Perceived benefits include an improvement in survival, reduction in local recurrence and downstaging of tumour burden.

8.5 Anti HER2 treatment

HER2 targeted immunotherapy consists of monoclonal antibodies (e.g., Trastuzumab)—previously discussed.

8.6 Other treatments

PARP inhibitors: poly ADP Ribose Polymerase inhibitors are targeted therapies with increasing use in patients with a PV in the *BRCA1/2* gene. This is discussed in more detail later.

Immunotherapy: this involves stimulating the host immune system actively immunisation (use of cancer vaccine) or passive immunisation (use of tumour specific antibodies or immune modulators). Of particular growing importance is the identification of patients with TNBC overexpressing immune evasion molecules (e.g., PDL: programmed death ligand) that may offer an additional treatment modality in this poor prognosis group [12].

9. Breast cancer genetics

The majority of breast cancers arise spontaneously—with known risk factors that include oestrogen exposure, reproductive history (late first or no pregnancy) and lifestyle practices. However, a significant proportion (20–30%) of cancers will have an inherited component, with family history remaining the strongest risk factor [13]. These tend to be classed as germline PVs in contrast to somatic mutations—arising from the interactions between environment and genetics.

Approximately 5–10% of breast cancer will have a strong inherited component that can be further sub-divided [13] according to strength of penetrance:

9.1 High penetrance genes

- *BRCA1*
- *BRCA2*
- *PALB2*

- *TP53*
- *PTEN*
- *STK11*
- *CDH1*

9.2 Moderate penetrance genes

- *ATM*
- *CHEK2*
- *NF1*
- *BARD1*

9.3 Low penetrance genes

The advent of Genome wide association studies has rapidly enabled the identification of over 100 breast cancer single nucleotide polymorphisms [14] that confer a small individual increase or decrease in breast cancer risk, but appear to work in a polygenic, multiplicative pattern contributing to a more significant risk.

10. Breast cancer and the *BRCA1* gene

This tumour suppressor gene was first identified in 1990 and cloned 4 years later in the US [15]. During the next two decades a bitter commercial battle ensued regarding patenting of the genomic DNA sequence to both *BRCA1* and *BRCA2*. Ultimately, the 2013 US Supreme Court (Association of Molecular Pathology vs. Myriad Genetics) ruled that "*isolation of genes found in nature do not render them patentable*" [16].

The human *BRCA1* gene (Chromosome 17—codes for the breast cancer type 1 susceptibility protein) is involved in non error prone homologous DNA repair. The majority of PVs are frameshift resulting in a truncated protein with founder PVs in the Ashkenazi Jewish populations and Eastern European population [13].

10.1 Penetrance and lifetime risk

The inheritance pattern is autosomal dominant with birth incidence of a *BRCA1* PV estimated at 1 in 500–900, accounting for 7–10% of familial breast cancer [13].

Harbouring a *BRCA1* PV confers a lifetime risk of breast cancer of approximately 60–85% [17, 18] and up to 60% for developing ovarian cancer (usually high-grade serous carcinomas). Risk of breast cancer is inversely proportional to age—a trend not so clearly seen in ovarian cancer (i.e., not age dependant). A recent prospective cohort study of 6036 *BRCA1* PV carriers [19] identified that the breast cancer incidences per decade of age increased from 21–30 years to 31–40 years but then remained at 23.5–28.3 per 1000 person years from age 31 to 70 years. Therefore, there is a rapid increase in breast cancer incidence in early childhood that plateaus and remains constant throughout the remaining adult life.

Family history of breast cancers amongst first and second-degree relatives increased the relative risk breast cancer, a trend not seen in ovarian cancer risk in families with ovarian cancer. *BRCA1* PVs located outside the region bounded by c.2282 to c.4071 were associated with the highest risk of developing breast cancer [19].

There is a significant risk of developing a contralateral breast cancer once diagnosed with breast cancer. Our own studies have confirmed that this risk is approximately 2–3% per year, persists for at least 30 years.

Other cancers associated with this PV include pancreatic cancer (RR 2.26), uterine body and cervical cancer (RR 2.65, RR 3.72, respectively) and prostate cancer in the under 65s (1.82) [13].

10.2 Pathology of *BRCA1* cancers

BRCA1 related breast cancers are heterogenous but have some important clinical features. They are most often triple negative approximately 70–80% (ER, PR, Her2 −ve) with expression of basal markers (CK5/6, CK14, SMA, P Cadherin, EGFR0). Histologically, they are similar to high-grade medullary carcinomas with pushing margins, high mitotic counts and lymphocytic infiltrate [20].

The international collaborative study (CIMBA) assessed pathological characteristics amongst 3797 *BRCA1* carriers [21] and identified that the mean age of breast cancer was 40 years. The majority of breast cancers were of the ductal, no-special type variety with the majority of cancers demonstrating a basal-triple negative phenotype (78% of tumours were ER-negative, 79% were PR-negative, 90% HER2-negative and 68% TNBC). High-grade tumours were most common, with a clear relationship between age at diagnosis and grade of breast cancer—grade decreased with increasing age.

11. Breast cancer and the *BRCA2* gene

This DNA repair gene was localised in the UK in 1994 and identified (cloned) in 1995 [22]. It is situated on Chromosome 13 at position 12.3 (13q12.3). Although the structures of the *BRCA1* and *BRCA2* gene vary from each other, there is some functional overlap. BRCA1 associates with *BRCA2* through *PALB2*, a major binding partner of BRCA2. There is some data to suggest that BRCA1 acts as an upstream regulator of *BRCA2* as *BRCA1* promotes the concentration of *PALB2* and *BRCA2* at DNA damage sites [23].

11.1 Penetrance and lifetime risk

PVs in *BRCA2* are nearly all inherited suggesting a large founder effect. This is important for practical purposes as certain populations can be tested for known PVs (e.g., single PV 999del5 accounts for almost all inherited breast and ovarian cancer in Iceland) [13].

Lifetime breast cancer risk has a wider range (40–85%) compared with *BRCA1*, and a slightly lower risk of developing ovarian cancer (20–30%) [13]. Approximately 1 in 400–800 women carry a PV (outbred population) that accounts for 10% of familial breast/ovarian cancer [14].

Several other cancers are more commonly associated with these PV: cholangiocarcinoma, melanoma, pancreatic cancer (overall RR 4.1), gastric cancer (RR 2.7) and prostate cancer (10–20% life time risk) [13]. Approximately 10% of male breast cancer is associated with *BRCA2*, a trend not seen in *BRCA1* PVs.

11.2 Pathology of *BRCA2* cancers

Breast cancer in *BRCA2* PVs carriers is a more heterogeneous group compared with *BRCA1* carriers, with more semblance to sporadic breast cancers. Pathology shows that these breast cancers are more often ER+ve compared with controls, with some studies showing increased DCIS and lobular cancer [20].

A study of breast cancer amongst 6893 *BRCA1* and *BRCA2* PV carriers found similar proportion of ductal, no-special type cancers (approximately 80%) with a four-fold increase in lobular cancers amongst *BRCA2* carriers (8% compared with 2% in *BRCA1* patients) [21]. Overall, there were double the number of Grade 1 and 2 cancers in the *BRCA2* compared with *BRCA1*, with more Grade 3 cancers in the *BRCA1* group (77% compared with 50% in *BRCA2* carriers).

There is paucity of data regarding the pre-invasive progression pathway amongst *BRCA1/2* carriers. Whereas a DCIS associated pre-malignant pathway has been postulated in sporadic cancers, this has not been shown in *BRCA1/2* PV carriers. There is conflicting data regarding incidence of DCIS in this patient group. Some reports suggest an increased incidence of DCIS identified in risk-reducing mastectomy specimens as opposed to other studies identifying DCIS less frequently near the invasive cancer compared with sporadic tumours [24].

12. Prognosis for *BRCA* mutated breast cancer

The POSH study (Prospective Outcomes in Sporadic versus Hereditary breast cancer), designed as a prospective cohort study, assessed the outcomes of women aged 40 years or below diagnosed with an invasive breast cancer in the UK [25]. With a follow up of nearly 10 years, 12% of all patients were identified with a PV in either the *BRCA1/2* gene. Multivariate analysis identified no overall difference in survival between *BRCA* positive or *BRCA* negative patients. Amongst patients with TNBC, there was a short-term survival benefit at 2 years amongst *BRCA* carriers. The authors hypothesised that this short-lived benefit may reflect greater sensitivity of BRCA mutant cancer to chemotherapy and/or greater visibility of BRCA related cancers to the immune system [25].

Studies prior to the POSH studied inconsistent effects of *BRCA1/2* PV status on breast cancer outcomes. A meta-analysis of 66 relevant studies [26] did not identify inferior breast cancer outcomes amongst *BRCA1/2* PV carriers despite the biological differences in breast cancer type already discussed.

In addition these women have similar survival whether they are treated with breast conservation surgery or a mastectomy, despite having significant higher rates of local failure with breast conservation [27]. An international longitudinal study of 655 patients with *BRCA1/2* PVs showed no differences in overall survival, distant or regional recurrence at 20 years whether women underwent a mastectomy or breast conservation therapy with radiotherapy. Interestingly, most local recurrences are second primary breast cancers rather than failure to control the primary breast cancer [27].

12.1 Radiotherapy

The effect of radiotherapy on *BRCA1/2* associated breast cancer merits consideration. These cancers are characterised by defects in homologous recombination, resulting in inadequate repair of double stranded DNA breaks—a hallmark of PVs in the *BRCA1/2* genes. In particular, younger patients with a higher rate of cell proliferation may be more susceptible to the carcinogenic effects of radiotherapy. Studies have confirmed an increased risk of contralateral breast cancer amongst young patients with a sporadic breast cancer treated with radiotherapy suggesting an effect of low-dose scatter radiation to surround healthy tissue [28].

In patients with a *BRCA1/2* PV associated breast cancer treated with unilateral radiotherapy, hypothetically there should be an increased risk of contralateral breast cancers particularly in the younger patient group, as the contralateral healthy breast will receive some scatter radiation. In addition, adjuvant radiotherapy to the index breast of *BRCA1/2* PV carriers should be more efficacious compared with sporadic cancer by virtue of the aberration in DNA repair. A recent Dutch study was not able to demonstrate any association between radiotherapy and contralateral breast cancer risk [29]. They observed a growing trend in their population group of *BRCA1/2* PV carriers away from breast conservation with radiotherapy towards mastectomy and contralateral mastectomy.

12.2 Chemotherapy

Healthy, normal breast tissue exposed to toxic, chemotherapeutic agents will result in DNA damage that is then partly repaired by the *BRCA1/2* DNA damage response. Different chemotherapy agents used to treat breast cancers exhibit differences in mechanism of action. Taxane-based agents work by disrupting the microtubule function whereas anthracyclines induce topoisomerase II mediated toxicity, DNA intercalation and generation of reactive oxidative species. In vitro studies have shown that platinum based chemotoxic agents have a greater sensitivity for *BRCA1* mutated cell lines which may in part be due to the disruption of DNA [30].

12.3 PARP inhibitors

This class of targeted therapy work on the principle of "synthetic lethality" [31], whereby a defect in one gene/protein results in cell survival however when synthesised with another gene/protein results in cell death.

Poly ADP Ribose Polymerase (PARP1) is an important protein that repairs single strand DNA breaks. Drugs that inhibit this protein (PARP inhibitors) result in multiple breaks in double stranded DNA that cannot be repaired, resulting in cell death. A proof of concept international study [32] showed a favourable therapeutic index for Olaparib (an orally active PARP inhibitor) amongst patients with advanced or recurrent breast cancer who harboured a *BRCA1/2* PV. The OlympiAD study, an international, randomised, Phase III trial recently reported an improved progression free survival amongst patients with metastatic breast cancer who were HER2 negative with a germline PV in either *BRCA1/2* [33]. Future directions of research will include combining PARP inhibitors with radiotherapy and platinum based agents [34].

12.4 Risk-reducing surgery

Bilateral risk-reducing mastectomy (BRRM) offers the greatest magnitude of overall risk reduction in health patients harboring a *BRCA1/2* PV by removing in excess of 90% of the breast tissue. A recent Cochrane review showed that BRRM reduces the risk of developing breast cancer by 85–100 [35] in high-risk patients. It also showed that BRRM reduced the risk of dying from breast cancer by 81–100% in high-risk patients and 100% in the moderate risk group.

Uptake of BRRM varies amongst women in this high-risk group. From a patient's perspective, young age and motherhood seem to be positive predictors for choosing surgery [36–38]. Several studies have shown international variations in uptake of BRRM with the highest rates in the UK and the Netherlands (33–50%) and the US (36%) compared with Poland (3%) and Israel (4%) [39, 40]. Differences in culture, healthcare systems and access to genetic testing are likely to contribute to these differences. However, wide variations are found within countries—for example in three different Canadian regions, the range of uptake was from 8 to 46% [41]—suggesting that other factors are important.

Media coverage and public interest in BRRM has been heightened since 2013 when Angelina Jolie's revealed her personal experience of bilateral mastectomies based on her inheriting a pathogenic *BRCA1* PV from her late mother. The so-called "Angelina Jolie Effect" ensued with increased uptake of genetic testing and BRRM in the US and UK [42–44].

12.5 Bilateral risk-reducing salpingo oophorectomy (BRRSO)

Women choosing this procedure will reduce their risk of developing ovarian by almost 90%. In addition, there appears to be a reduction in their subsequent risk of developing breast cancer (premenopausal women) [45, 46], with several previous studies showing a risk-reduction of almost 50%. Unlike breast cancer, surveillance for ovarian cancer is limited to measurements of tumour markers (CA125) and transvaginal ultra-sound—both of which may lack sensitivity. As such, uptake of BRRSO is high (up to 75%).

BRRSO renders women post menopausal (surgical menopause) with additional risks to the cardiovascular and skeletal system. In addition, most women are recommended to have completed their family prior to considering this surgery. The climacteric symptoms following this procedure can be debilitating and many women will consider use of HRT to combat these symptoms. Use of HRT itself may increase the risk of developing breast cancer in these women already deemed at high-risk.

The risk reduction for breast cancer has recently been reassessed for potential selection bias [47]. This study used the same methodology previously described [45] to study a cohort of Dutch *BRCA1/2* healthy carriers and found that following BRRSO, the incidence of breast cancer was almost halved (Hazard Ratio 0.36–0.62). A revised analysis taking into account the various biases described above showed no real protective effect of BRRSO on breast cancer development (Hazard Ratio 1.09). This has important clinical implications when considering the variations of uptake of BRRM compared with BRRSO—women only choosing BRRSO over BRRM may have had their breast cancer risk reduction overestimated if they only chose BRRSO.

12.6 Chemoprevention

In the UK, healthy women with a *BRCA1/2* PV may consider three medications to reduce their risk:

Tamoxifen: this selective oestrogen receptor modulator (first generation) has been shown to reduce the risk in asymptomatic women by approximately 40–50% [48]. In women with breast cancer, tamoxifen has a similar risk reduction in developing CBC. The side-effect profile (hot flushes, increased incidence of endometrial cancer, thromboembolic phenomenon) is an important consideration as less than 15% of women will choose this and remain compliant [49]. Tamoxifen may be considered in pre and post menopausal women.

Raloxifene (second generation SERM), used in the prevention and treatment of osteoporosis has a much better side effect profile with no increase in endometrial cancers but increases thromboembolic risk similar to tamoxifen. Risk reduction was inferior to tamoxifen over an extended follow [50]. Raloxifene is considered in the post-menopausal setting only.

Aromatase inhibitor: Exemestane has been shown to offer 65% relative risk reduction in post-menopausal women at increased risk with a minimal side-effect profile [51]. The IBIS II trial (International Breast Cancer Intervention Studies) randomised post-menopausal women with an increased risk of breast cancer to anastrozole or placebo. At 5 years follow-up, 2% of women taking Anastrozole had developed breast cancer compared with 4% in the placebo group [52].

Although there is not good quality evidence to show that endocrine therapy is not effective in *BRCA1* as 70–80% of breast cancers are triple negative and these medications only reduce ER positive cancers they may have less efficacy in *BRCA1* PV carriers.

12.7 Lifestyle

Worldwide, the number of oestrogen receptor positive breast cancers is increasing with a reverse pattern seen with oestrogen negative cancer. In developed countries, hormone sensitive breast cancer is particularly amenable to lifestyle prevention—with recent studies suggesting that modification of lifestyle measure may prevent up to 30% of breast cancers [53].

Amongst *BRCA* carriers, smoking, increased weight and reduced physical activity further increases the risk of breast cancer. These lifestyle measures need to commence in adolescence and adherence to this (150 min weekly activity, BMI < 25, <1 alcoholic drink daily) has been shown to reduce mortality in *BRCA* carriers by almost 60% [54].

The LIBRE study (Lifestyle Intervention in *BRCA1/2* PV carriers) aims to randomise healthy *BRCA1/2* PV carriers to a number of lifestyles interventions versus a control group and assess changes in physical and psychological well being [55].

13. Discussion

The worldwide burden of breast cancer poses significant challenges to health care providers. There is an increasing awareness that this heterogenous disease requires a multi-modality approach with consideration to both prevention and treatment.

Diet and lifestyle are important modifiers in the prevention of breast cancer. Adherence to physical activity and alcohol guidelines may reduce the risk of developing breast cancer (pre and post menopausal), with weight control being more important in prevention in the post menopausal cohort [56]. Energy restriction, in particular intermittently is association with changes in breast gene expression and systemic metabolism [57]. Future studies will need to assess the mechanism and clinical significance in breast cancer pathogenesis.

Breast cancer metabolomics is an area of growing interest. A recent study was able to determine a differential metabolic signature based on *BRCA1* functionality [58] and may provide future biomarkers.

An area of interest is establishing whether breast cancer may be considered a communicable disease. There is established causality of infection with the Human Papilloma Virus and a number of cancers namely cervical cancer and associations with penile, anal and vulvar cancer. A similar aetiology has been postulated with breast cancer with entry of the virus via the nipple areolar complex resulting in biological activity within the mammary duct epithelium resulting in breast cancer. Data from Norway [59] have identified a possible association of pre-malignant changes in the cervix and an increased risk of subsequent breast cancer. A subsequent UK study [60] has identified the presence of high-risk HPV DNA in 42% of breast cancers with viral activity confirmed in less than 20% of invasive cancers suggesting that this may be an area of on going interest in the future.

Gene therapy in cancer aims at correcting specific genetic anomalies contributing to the development of certain cancers. This can be subdivided into germline and somatic cell gene therapy and is an important treatment modality in disease processes like cystic fibrosis and blood disorders. Several *BRCA1* retroviral vectors were

DOI: http://dx.doi.org/10.5772/intechopen.90926

assessed in Phase 2 clinical trials in ovarian cancer almost two decades ago [61] with some initial potential as a therapeutic modality. The lack of progress in viral vectors suggests that newer techniques such as gene editing may find a place.

The UK 100,000 Genome project completed recruitment in 2018. Breast cancer patients represent a significant proportion of the 85,000 patients either with a cancer or rare disease diagnosis. Whole genome sequencing has allowed rapid analysis of the entire genome in this patient subgroup and is already aiding clinicians in making therapeutic decision in breast cancer, although no new hereditary genes have yet been identified from this initiative.

14. Conclusion

Pathogenic variants in the *BRCA1* and *BRCA2* gene confer a substantial lifetime risk of developing breast cancer. These breast cancers display characteristic clinical and pathological features that are important in the clinical management of the disease.

Multiple strategies exist for healthy individuals harbouring PVs in these genes. This comprises surveillance using modern day radiology (mammography and MRI scans) and risk reducing strategies. The latter include bilateral risk-reducing mastectomy, bilateral salpingo-oophorectomy, chemoprevention and lifestyle modification.

Author details

Naren Basu[1,2]* and D. Gareth Evans[3,4]

1 University Hospitals Birmingham, UK

2 University of Birmingham, UK

3 University of Manchester, Manchester, UK

4 Central Manchester Hospitals NHS Foundation Trust and The Christie NHS Foundation Trust, Manchester, UK

*Address all correspondence to: naren_basu@hotmail.com

References

[1] World Cancer Research Fund. Breast Cancer Statistics. 2018. Available from: https://www.wcrf.org/dietandcancer/cancer-trends/breast-cancer-statistics

[2] Cancer Research UK. Breast Cancer. 2019. Available from: https://www.cancerresearchuk.org/about-cancer/breast-cancer/about

[3] Union for International Cancer Control. New Global Cancer Data: GLOBOCAN 2018. 2019. Available from: https://www.uicc.org/news/new-global-cancer-data-globocan-2018

[4] van der Borden CL, Stoffers S, Lips EH, Wesseling J. Avoiding overtreatment of ductal carcinoma in situ. Trends in Cancer. 2019;**5**(7):391-393

[5] Makki J. Diversity of breast carcinoma: Histological subtypes and clinical relevance. Clinical Medicine Insights: Pathology. 2015;**8**:23-31

[6] Lakhani S, Ellis I, Schnitt S, Tan P, van de Vijver M. WHO Classification of Breast Tumors. Lyon: IARC; 2012

[7] Love RR, Philips J. Oophorectomy for breast cancer: History revisited. JNCI: Journal of the National Cancer Institute. 2002;**94**(19):1433-1434

[8] Murphy CG, Dickler MN. Endocrine resistance in hormone-responsive breast cancer: Mechanisms and therapeutic strategies. Endocrine-Related Cancer. 2016;**23**(8):R337-R352

[9] Hudis CA. Trastuzumab—Mechanism of action and use in clinical practice. The New England Journal of Medicine. 2007;**357**(1):39-51

[10] Fragomeni SM, Sciallis A, Jeruss JS. Molecular subtypes and local-regional control of breast cancer. Surgical Oncology Clinics of North America. 2018;**27**(1):95-120

[11] Fisher B, Anderson S, Bryant J, Margolese RG, Deutsch M, Fisher ER, et al. Twenty-year follow-up of a randomized trial comparing total mastectomy, lumpectomy, and lumpectomy plus irradiation for the treatment of invasive breast cancer. The New England Journal of Medicine. 2002;**347**(16):1233-1241

[12] Marra A, Viale G, Curigliano G. Recent advances in triple negative breast cancer: The immunotherapy era. BMC Medicine. 2019;**17**(1):90

[13] Lalloo F, Evans DG. Familial breast cancer. Clinical Genetics. 2012;**82**(2):105-114

[14] Mavaddat N, Peock S, Frost D, Ellis S, Platte R, Fineberg E, et al. Cancer risks for BRCA1 and BRCA2 mutation carriers: Results from prospective analysis of EMBRACE. Journal of the National Cancer Institute. 2013;**105**(11):812-822

[15] Claus EB, Risch N, Thompson WD. Genetic analysis of breast cancer in the cancer and steroid hormone study. American Journal of Human Genetics. 1991;**48**(2):232-242

[16] Sherkow JS, Greely HT. The history of patenting genetic material. Annual Review of Genetics. 2015;**49**:161-182

[17] Evans DG, Shenton A, Woodward E, Lalloo F, Howell A, Maher ER. Penetrance estimates for BRCA1 and BRCA2 based on genetic testing in a Clinical Cancer Genetics service setting: Risks of breast/ovarian cancer quoted should reflect the cancer burden in the family. BMC Cancer. 2008;**8**:155

[18] Ford D, Easton DF, Stratton M, Narod S, Goldgar D, Devilee P, et al.

Genetic heterogeneity and penetrance analysis of the BRCA1 and BRCA2 genes in breast cancer families. The Breast Cancer Linkage Consortium. American Journal of Human Genetics. 1998;**62**(3):676-689

[19] Kuchenbaecker KB, Hopper JL, Barnes DR, Phillips KA, Mooij TM, Roos-Blom MJ, et al. Risks of breast, ovarian, and contralateral breast cancer for BRCA1 and BRCA2 mutation carriers. JAMA. 2017;**317**(23):2402-2416

[20] Da Silva L, Lakhani SR. Pathology of hereditary breast cancer. Modern Pathology. 2010;**23**(Suppl 2):S46-S51

[21] Mavaddat N, Barrowdale D, Andrulis IL, Domchek SM, Eccles D, Nevanlinna H, et al. Pathology of breast and ovarian cancers among BRCA1 and BRCA2 mutation carriers: Results from the Consortium of Investigators of Modifiers of BRCA1/2 (CIMBA). Cancer Epidemiology, Biomarkers & Prevention. 2012;**21**(1):134-147

[22] Wooster R, Neuhausen SL, Mangion J, Quirk Y, Ford D, Collins N, et al. Localization of a breast cancer susceptibility gene, BRCA2, to chromosome 13q12-13. Science. 1994;**265**(5181):2088-2090

[23] Zhang F, Ma J, Wu J, Ye L, Cai H, Xia B, et al. PALB2 links BRCA1 and BRCA2 in the DNA-damage response. Current Biology: CB. 2009;**19**(6):524-529

[24] Yang RL, Mick R, Lee K, Graves HL, Nathanson KL, Domchek SM, et al. DCIS in BRCA1 and BRCA2 mutation carriers: Prevalence, phenotype, and expression of oncodrivers C-MET and HER3. Journal of Translational Medicine. 2015;**13**:335

[25] Copson ER, Maishman TC, Tapper WJ, Cutress RI, Greville-Heygate S, Altman DG, et al. Germline BRCA mutation and outcome in young-onset breast cancer (POSH): A prospective cohort study. The Lancet Oncology. 2018;**19**(2):169-180

[26] van den Broek AJ, Schmidt MK, van 't Veer LJ, Tollenaar RA, van Leeuwen FE. Worse breast cancer prognosis of BRCA1/BRCA2 mutation carriers: What's the evidence? A systematic review with meta-analysis. PLoS ONE. 2015;**10**(3):e0120189

[27] Pierce LJ, Phillips KA, Griffith KA, Buys S, Gaffney DK, Moran MS, et al. Local therapy in BRCA1 and BRCA2 mutation carriers with operable breast cancer: Comparison of breast conservation and mastectomy. Breast Cancer Research and Treatment. 2010;**121**(2):389-398

[28] Gao X, Fisher SG, Emami B. Risk of second primary cancer in the contralateral breast in women treated for early-stage breast cancer: A population-based study. International Journal of Radiation Oncology, Biology, Physics. 2003;**56**(4):1038-1045

[29] Drooger J, Akdeniz D, Pignol JP, Koppert LB, McCool D, Seynaeve CM, et al. Adjuvant radiotherapy for primary breast cancer in BRCA1 and BRCA2 mutation carriers and risk of contralateral breast cancer with special attention to patients irradiated at younger age. Breast Cancer Research and Treatment. 2015;**154**(1):171-180

[30] Tassone P, Tagliaferri P, Perricelli A, Blotta S, Quaresima B, Martelli ML, et al. BRCA1 expression modulates chemosensitivity of BRCA1-defective HCC1937 human breast cancer cells. British Journal of Cancer. 2003;**88**(8):1285-1291

[31] Lord CJ, Tutt AN, Ashworth A. Synthetic lethality and cancer therapy: Lessons learned from the development of PARP inhibitors. Annual Review of Medicine. 2015;**66**:455-470

[32] Tutt A, Robson M, Garber JE, Domchek SM, Audeh MW, Weitzel JN, et al. Oral poly(ADP-ribose) polymerase inhibitor olaparib in patients with BRCA1 or BRCA2 mutations and advanced breast cancer: A proof-of-concept trial. Lancet. 2010;**376**(9737):235-244

[33] Robson M, Im SA, Senkus E, Xu B, Domchek SM, Masuda N, et al. Olaparib for metastatic breast cancer in patients with a germline BRCA mutation. The New England Journal of Medicine. 2017;**377**(6):523-533

[34] Lee A, Moon BI, Kim TH. BRCA1/BRCA2 pathogenic variant breast cancer: Treatment and prevention strategies. Annals of Laboratory Medicine. 2020;**40**(2):114-121

[35] Lostumbo L, Carbine NE, Wallace J. Prophylactic mastectomy for the prevention of breast cancer. Cochrane Database of Systematic Reviews. 2010;**11**:CD002748

[36] Meijers-Heijboer EJ, Verhoog LC, Brekelmans CT, Seynaeve C, Tilanus-Linthorst MM, Wagner A, et al. Presymptomatic DNA testing and prophylactic surgery in families with a BRCA1 or BRCA2 mutation. Lancet. 2000;**355**(9220):2015-2020

[37] Evans DG, Baildam AD, Anderson E, Brain A, Shenton A, Vasen HF, et al. Risk reducing mastectomy: Outcomes in 10 European centres. Journal of Medical Genetics. 2009;**46**(4):254-258

[38] Evans DG, Lalloo F, Ashcroft L, Shenton A, Clancy T, Baildam AD, et al. Uptake of risk-reducing surgery in unaffected women at high risk of breast and ovarian cancer is risk, age, and time dependent. Cancer Epidemiology, Biomarkers & Prevention. 2009;**18**(8):2318-2324

[39] Den Heijer M, van Asperen CJ, Harris H, Nippert I, Schmidtke J, Bouhnik AD, et al. International variation in physicians' attitudes towards prophylactic mastectomy—Comparison between France, Germany, the Netherlands and the United Kingdom. European Journal of Cancer. 2013;**49**(13): 2798-2805

[40] Metcalfe KA, Birenbaum-Carmeli D, Lubinski J, Gronwald J, Lynch H, Moller P, et al. International variation in rates of uptake of preventive options in BRCA1 and BRCA2 mutation carriers. International Journal of Cancer. 2008;**122**(9):2017-2022

[41] Metcalfe KA, Ghadirian P, Rosen B, Foulkes W, Kim-Sing C, Eisen A, et al. Variation in rates of uptake of preventive options by Canadian women carrying the BRCA1 or BRCA2 genetic mutation. Open Medicine. 2007;**1**(2):e92-e98

[42] Liede A, Cai M, Crouter TF, Niepel D, Callaghan F, Evans DG. Risk-reducing mastectomy rates in the US: A closer examination of the Angelina Jolie effect. Breast Cancer Research and Treatment. 2018;**171**(2):435-442

[43] Evans DG, Barwell J, Eccles DM, Collins A, Izatt L, Jacobs C, et al. The Angelina Jolie effect: How high celebrity profile can have a major impact on provision of cancer related services. Breast Cancer Research. 2014;**16**(5):442

[44] Evans DG, Wisely J, Clancy T, Lalloo F, Wilson M, Johnson R, et al. Longer term effects of the Angelina Jolie effect: Increased risk-reducing mastectomy rates in BRCA carriers and other high-risk women. Breast Cancer Research. 2015;**17**:143

[45] Domchek SM, Friebel TM, Singer CF, Evans DG, Lynch HT, Isaacs C, et al. Association of risk-reducing surgery in BRCA1 or BRCA2

mutation carriers with cancer risk and mortality. JAMA. 2010;**304**(9):967-975

[46] Rebbeck TR, Lynch HT, Neuhausen SL, Narod SA, Van't Veer L, Garber JE, et al. Prophylactic oophorectomy in carriers of BRCA1 or BRCA2 mutations. The New England Journal of Medicine. 2002;**346**(21):1616-1622

[47] Heemskerk-Gerritsen BA, Seynaeve C, van Asperen CJ, Ausems MG, Collee JM, van Doorn HC, et al. Breast cancer risk after salpingo-oophorectomy in healthy BRCA1/2 mutation carriers: Revisiting the evidence for risk reduction. Journal of the National Cancer Institute. 2015;**107**(5)djv033:1-9

[48] Howell A, Anderson AS, Clarke RB, Duffy SW, Evans DG, Garcia-Closas M, et al. Risk determination and prevention of breast cancer. Breast Cancer Research. 2014;**16**(5):446

[49] Taylor R, Taguchi K. Tamoxifen for breast cancer chemoprevention: Low uptake by high-risk women after evaluation of a breast lump. Annals of Family Medicine. 2005;**3**(3):242-247

[50] Vogel VG, Costantino JP, Wickerham DL, Cronin WM, Cecchini RS, Atkins JN, et al. Effects of tamoxifen vs raloxifene on the risk of developing invasive breast cancer and other disease outcomes: The NSABP Study of Tamoxifen and Raloxifene (STAR) P-2 trial. JAMA. 2006;**295**(23):2727-2741

[51] Goss PE, Ingle JN, Ales-Martinez JE, Cheung AM, Chlebowski RT, Wactawski-Wende J, et al. Exemestane for breast-cancer prevention in postmenopausal women. The New England Journal of Medicine. 2011;**364**(25):2381-2391

[52] Cuzick J, Sestak I, Baum M, Buzdar A, Howell A, Dowsett M, et al. Effect of anastrozole and tamoxifen as adjuvant treatment for early-stage breast cancer: 10-year analysis of the ATAC trial. The Lancet Oncology. 2010;**11**(12):1135-1141

[53] Parkin DM, Boyd L, Walker LC. 16. The fraction of cancer attributable to lifestyle and environmental factors in the UK in 2010. British Journal of Cancer. 2011;**105**(Suppl 2):S77-S81

[54] Cloud AJ, Thai A, Liao Y, Terry MB. The impact of cancer prevention guideline adherence on overall mortality in a high-risk cohort of women from the New York site of the Breast Cancer Family Registry. Breast Cancer Research and Treatment. 2015;**149**(2):537-546

[55] Kiechle M, Engel C, Berling A, Hebestreit K, Bischoff SC, Dukatz R, et al. Effects of lifestyle intervention in BRCA1/2 mutation carriers on nutrition, BMI, and physical fitness (LIBRE study): Study protocol for a randomized controlled trial. Trials. 2016;**17**:368

[56] Harvie M, Howell A, Evans DG. Can diet and lifestyle prevent breast cancer: What is the evidence? American Society of Clinical Oncology Educational Book. 2015;**35**:e66-e73

[57] Harvie MN, Sims AH, Pegington M, Spence K, Mitchell A, Vaughan AA, et al. Intermittent energy restriction induces changes in breast gene expression and systemic metabolism. Breast Cancer Research. 2016;**18**(1):57

[58] Roig B, Rodriguez-Balada M, Samino S, Lam EW, Guaita-Esteruelas S, Gomes AR, et al. Metabolomics reveals novel blood plasma biomarkers associated to the BRCA1-mutated phenotype of human breast cancer. Scientific Reports. 2017;**7**(1):17831

[59] Hansen BT, Nygard M, Falk RS, Hofvind S. Breast cancer and ductal carcinoma in situ among women with prior squamous or glandular

precancer in the cervix: A register-based study. British Journal of Cancer. 2012;**107**(9):1451-1453

[60] Salman NA, Davies G, Majidy F, Shakir F, Akinrinade H, Perumal D, et al. Association of high risk human papillomavirus and breast cancer: A UK based study. Scientific Reports. 2017;7:43591

[61] Obermiller PS, Tait DL, Holt JT. Gene therapy for carcinoma of the breast: Therapeutic genetic correction strategies. Breast Cancer Research. 2000;**2**(1):28-31

Chapter 4

Epidemiology and Genetic Susceptibility of Breast and Ovarian Cancer in Sardinian Population

Grazia Palomba, Giuseppe Palmieri, Antonio Cossu, Panagiotis Paliogiannis and Maria Cristina Sini

Abstract

The objective of this population-based study is to describe epidemiological and genetic features of breast and ovarian cancer in North Sardinia, Italy. Patients who carry a high-risk mutation in one or both of the BRCA genes (BRCA1 or BRCA2) have a significantly increased risk of developing breast/ovarian cancer (BOC) and other cancers (e.g., prostate cancer in male). Epidemiological data on incidence distribution of breast/ovarian cancer from 2016 to 2019 in North Sardinia are obtained from the local tumor registry and from the cumulative results of 209 genetic testing for BRCA gene mutations performed in all young breast cancer patients and all women (over 50 years) with family history of BOC (total of 164 cases); further, 45 genetic testing is performed, on ovarian cancer patients, at any age. The results provide a different distribution of fraction mutations carried by women and a higher prevalence of the BRCA2 mutation in the north of Sardinia than the entire population and highlight the presence of specific germline mutation associated with the "founder effect" in distinct genetic subgroups reflecting genetic drift. Advances in next-generation sequencing technology, data analysis, and clinical investigation have revolutionized efforts to identify potential targets for BRCA molecular-based therapeutic agents.

Keywords: BRCA1, BRCA2, genetic epidemiology, genetic testing, founder mutations, breast cancer (BC), ovarian cancer (OC), breast and ovarian cancer syndrome (BOC)

1. Introduction

Breast cancer (BC) is the second most common cancer in the female world population, with more than 1.3 million new cases every year [1]. Systemic treatment of breast cancer is based on accurate knowledge of the clinical and molecular characteristics of the tumor and includes cytotoxic, hormonal, or biological agents. Therapies are used in the adjuvant, neo-adjuvant, and metastatic settings of BC patients. In general, systemic agents are active at the beginning of therapy in 90% of primary breast cancers and 50% of metastases. However, disease progression and resistance to therapy are expected to occur in a variable period of time, though they are becoming a less common event.

Ovarian cancer (OC) is the seventh most common cancer in women from Western countries (about 5% of all cancers) [2]; its frequency however varies widely among different geographic regions and ethnic groups, with a high incidence in Northern Europe and the United States and low rates in Africa and Asia. In Europe, about 61,000 new cases are estimated to be diagnosed per year. The age-adjusted world incidence is around 11 new cases per 100,000 inhabitants per year.

The majority of OC cases are sporadic, and only 5–10% of them are familial. Ovarian cancer is usually diagnosed at an advanced stage and etiology remains poorly understood. Nevertheless, about 30% of patients present with early-stage disease (FIGO stage I–IIA). Surgery plays a main role in the treatment of epithelial ovarian cancer, and an extensive surgical staging is crucial in selecting the most appropriate systemic therapy. Several factors are associated with the onset of the epithelial ovarian cancer, including age (it is a disease of older age), genetic features (approximately, 5–10% of them result from a hereditary predisposition), site-specific ovarian cancer syndrome (10–15% of all cases), and a positive family history with an affected first-degree relative (mother, daughter, or sister).

In the presence of the breast-ovarian cancer syndrome (BOC), families present with multiple cases (two or more) affected by ovarian and breast cancer in successive generations, tumors with earlier age of onset (usually in the premenopausal age), and evidence of both maternal and paternal transmission [3]. This hereditary syndrome has been linked to the BRCA1 gene at chromosome 17q12–21 (81% of cases) and, less frequently, to the BRCA2 gene at chromosome 13q.

Cumulative breast cancer risks by age 70 are estimated to be 65% for BRCA1 and 45% for BRCA2 mutation carriers. In addition, women with BRCA mutations are at significant risk of developing ovarian cancer and other malignancies [4].

Both *BRCA1* and *BRCA2* encode proteins that are involved in maintenance of genome stability and in the repair of double-stranded DNA breaks (DSBs) by homologous recombination (HR).

HR is a potentially error-free mechanism of DNA damage repair that requires RAD51 localization to DSBs. BRCA2 interacts directly with RAD51 and is required for the formation of RAD51 complex, as is a BRCA2-associated protein called DSS1. The BRCA2 protein contains several copies of a 70 aa motif called the BRC motif, and these motifs mediate binding to the RAD51 recombinase, which functions in DNA repair. BRCA2 is considered a tumor suppressor gene, as tumors with BRCA2 mutations generally exhibit loss of heterozygosity (LOH) of the wild-type allele. BRCA1 is also required for the formation of RAD51 foci, perhaps through direct or indirect interaction with RAD51 or BRCA2 [5]. *BRCA2* has also been identified as the *FANCD1* gene, a member of the Fanconi anemia complex of proteins, and cells deficient in this protein have a similar phenotype to those deficient in BRCA [6]. Chromosomal instability as a result of BRCA1 or BRCA2 deficiency may be the pathogenic basis for breast tumor formation. In women who inherit an inactivating mutation, BRCA deficiency is critical to the development of disease and is the result of both the inherited inactivating allele and somatic genomic loss of the wild-type allele in breast or ovarian epithelial cells. The risk of developing BRCA-associated ovarian cancer is modified by several factors such as the reproductive history and hormonal exposure of an affected individual, and the coinheritance of modifying genes [6].

2. Breast ovarian cancer family selection

The overall criteria to reconstruct the possible family history of patients with breast cancer can be established by identifying three risk levels: profile 1, level of cancer risk equivalent to general population; profile 2, level of cancer risk two-fold higher than that of general population; and profile 3, level of cancer risk three or more times higher than that of general population.

Six main criteria are taken into consideration to address women diagnosed with breast cancer into the general population to BRCA mutation testing: (a) younger women with breast cancer diagnosed at age less than 36 years; (b) affected male individuals (at any age of onset); (c) women with occurrence of both breast and ovarian cancer (at any age); (d) women with bilateral carcinoma diagnosed before 50 years; (e) women with triple-negative breast cancer who are younger than 50 years; and (f) all women with ovarian (and fallopian tube) carcinoma before 50 years or with high-grade serous ovarian cancer at any age.

Current guidelines recommend genetic testing for women diagnosed with breast cancer and at least one affected family member; a personal history of breast cancer and one or more relatives with breast cancer diagnosed before age 50; two or more relatives diagnosed with breast cancer at any age; one or more relatives with ovarian cancer; one or more relatives with male breast cancer, or two or more relatives with prostate cancer or pancreatic cancer.

In this sense, the American Society of Clinical Oncology, the American College of Obstetrics and Gynecology, and the National Comprehensive Cancer Network do not recommend BRCA mutation testing for women younger than 50 years with breast cancer unless there is a family history of breast/ovarian cancer [7, 8]. Therefore, many young women with breast cancer and lack of a family history of disease will not have the opportunity to undergo BRCA mutation testing. As a result of this, a significant proportion of newly diagnosed women with breast cancer who are younger than 50 years may not be identified as BRCA mutation carriers, and they remain at high risk for subsequent breast and ovarian cancer. Positive BRCA mutation testing in women with ovarian carcinoma allows relatives access to oncological genetic counseling and preventive testing, aimed at verifying the presence or absence in family members, of pathogenic sequence variants. Genetic results are essential to carry out specific recommendations for clinical management of at-risk relatives. In the case of a positive result, the programs are aimed at promoting screening strategies for early diagnosis as well as favoring primary prevention interventions for the reduction in the risk of breast/ovarian cancer. The BRCA test is recommended for all patients with nonmucinous and nonborderline ovarian cancer, carcinoma of the fallopian tubes, or peritoneal primitive carcinoma. It is important to offer the BRCA test since cancer diagnosis. The identification of a pathogenic variant in BRCA genes also allows patients to plan an adequate therapeutic pathway. The identification of pathogenic variant in BRCA genes at germinal level in a patient with ovarian cancer allows to undertake a path of oncogenetic counseling in family members in order to identify high-risk carriers and to propose targeted programs for early diagnosis of syndrome-associated tumors with BRCA-related and to carry out strategies aimed at reducing the risk.

In BRCA-mutated women, with ascertained diagnosis of ovarian cancer, a psychosocial approach must be envisaged, which takes into account the impact of the diagnosis and treatment on the physical and psycho-emotional sphere, as well as the psychological implications of the hereditary problem and the involvement of healthy family members at risk in the decision-making process [9].

2.1 BRCA molecular profiling and epidemiology in Sardinia population

In Sardinia, breast cancer represents the principal death-causing malignancy, with an incidence similar to that observed in western countries [10]. Familial aggregation is thought to account for 5–10% of all breast cancer cases, and germline mutations in different genes involved in pathways critical to maintain the genomic integrity have accounted for less than 25% of the inherited breast cancer. Prevalence of mutation carriers with breast or ovarian cancer depends on the population studied and displays considerable variation based on ethnic and geographical diversity [11]. In Italy, 4–27% of the identified mutations recurred among apparently unrelated families, while a regional founder effect has been demonstrated for few mutations; contribution of BRCA1–2 mutations to breast cancer predisposition has been reported for populations from the Northern part of Sardinia as well as strong founder effects for several genetic diseases were founded with some geographical differences within the island [12]. BRCA2 mutations are notably more recurrent than BRCA1 mutations in breast cancer families from North Sardinia [13]. Moreover, allelic transmission is identical in males and females as the entire population should comply with the Hardy–Weinberg law [14].

In southern Italy, including Sardinia, standardized mortality rate in ovarian cancer patients is 8.5/100,000 lower than in Italy; also, the cumulative risk of death from the disease is extremely low (0.4%) [4, 15].

Germline mutations in either BRCA1 or BRCA2 genes occur in approximately 10% of unselected women with ovarian cancer, and women with inherited BRCA1/2 mutations are at significant risk of developing ovarian cancer [16].

The lifetime risk of developing ovarian cancer in women who carry a germline BRCA mutation has been estimated to be of 40–60% for BRCA1 and 11–27% for BRCA2 [17]. A meta-analysis of 22 studies with over 8000 disease probands has defined the incidence for ovarian cancer to be approximately 39% for BRCA1 and 11% for BRCA2 [18]. In North Sardinia, less than 10% of breast cancer families presented an association with ovarian cancer (at least one affected family member) [12]. Nevertheless, the presence of ovarian cancer was demonstrated to significantly increase the occurrence of BRCA1/2 germline mutations in Sardinian breast cancer families [12, 19].

2.2 Next-generation sequencing approaches for mutation analyses in Sardinian population

In recent past years, epidemiological data have become available from the Cancer Registry of the Province of Sassari. This registry was created in 1992 by the Local Health Agency (Azienda Sanitaria Locale, ASL) of Sassari for the epidemiological surveillance of tumors in the province. In 1999, it became part of wider web tumor registries, coordinated today by the Italian Association for Tumor Registries (Associazione Italiana Registri Tumori) [20]. Crude incidence and mortality rates for 100,000 inhabitants per year were calculated and standardized rates adjusted for European age population standards. The age-class distribution of cases was analyzed; relative incidence and mortality date was compared between Sardinia and the rest of Italy (**Table 1**).

Numerous studies by our group have assessed the BRCA1/2 mutation prevalence in various cohorts, although few have evaluated the predictors for the occurrence of both BRCA1 and BRCA2 mutations among younger patients in a hospital-based population.

Breast/ovarian cancer patients, originating from North Sardinia, were recruited from clinics at the University of Sassari and Local Health Agencies accounting for cancer patients from the Central and Northern part of the island (Sassari, Olbia,

Age class	No. of cases	% of cases
A: age-class incidence distribution of breast cancer cases (N = 164) in North Sardinia, 2016–2019		
0–14	—	—
15–29	2	1.2
30–40	37	22.5
40–50	53	32.3
*50+	72	43.9
B: age-class incidence distribution of ovarian cancer cases (N = 45) in North Sardinia, 2016–2019		
0–14	—	—
15–29	—	—
30–44	4	8.9
45–59	17	37.8
60–74	18	40
75+	6	13.3

Asterisk indicates familial breast cancer patients.

Table 1.
Epidemiological data in North Sardinia.

Nuoro). Sardinian origin was ascertained in all cases through genealogical studies. Patients with a histologically-proven diagnosis of breast/ovarian cancer diagnosed before 50 years were consecutively-collected during a period of 4 years; no additional selection criteria were used for their inclusion into the study.

In such a population-based series of early-onset breast/ovarian cancer, family history of breast and ovarian cancers were assessed according to the above-described standardized criteria. Patients were informed of the aims of the study and blood samples were obtained with their written consent. Genomic DNA was isolated and next-generation sequencing (NGS) investigations were performed using a specific BRCA1/2 gene. Research assay panel allows to detect simultaneously point mutations and CNVs. Samples were sequenced on the Ion Torrent S5 System (Life Technologies, Waltham, MA, USA), and data were processed with the Ion Torrent platform.

Between 2016 and 2019, 209 patients originating from North Sardinia underwent the NGS-based mutation analyzed in BRCA1/2 genes; among them, 164 were diagnosed with primary breast cancer and 45 with primary ovarian cancer, with median age at onset of 51 years (range 27 ± 84), any age for ovarian cancer.

Patients with first diagnosis of breast cancer were evaluated for familial occurrence of malignancy using a questionnaire to interview probands about their first- and second-degree relatives. In our series of Sardinian cases, we analyzed sporadic young patients with a breast cancer diagnosis before 50 years (59/164; 36%) and any familiar history; a number of probands with a positive family history for breast cancer (33/164; 20%) and age of onset before 50 years; and patients (72/164; 44%) with breast/ovarian cancer familiar history at any age. Moreover, the analysis was performed on 45 (45/209; 21.5%) ovarian cases at any age.

2.3 Deleterious variants in BRCA1 and BRCA2 genes

Overall, prevalence of deleterious BRCA1/2 variants was 10 times higher in patients with a positive family history (19/105; 18.09%) as compared with those with sporadic tumors (2/104; 1.92%). Interestingly, all uncertain variants-that is, those with unknown functional significance-were nearly completely prevalent in familiar tumor cases. Deleterious variants were found in 68% (15/22) of breast cancer cases and 31.8% (7/22) of ovarian cancer cases; variants with unknown significance (VUS) were observed in 81.2% of breast cancer patients and in 18.7% of ovarian cancer patients. Deleterious germline variants in BRCA2 5.74% (12/209) were featured, followed by BRCA1 4.78%(10/209) patients according to our previous study that explained a different geographical distribution of BRCA1–2 mutations with a higher prevalence of the BRCA2 mutation in the north of Sardinia than the entire population [19].

Among families with high recurrence of breast cancer ($\geq$ 3 cases in first-degree relatives), almost all ones from northern Sardinia were previously demonstrated by our group to share the same haplotype and carry a single mutation in BRCA2 gene (BRCA2-8765delAG), which thus acts as a pathogenic variant with founder effect in the population of this part of the island (due to the occurrence and propagation of a common ancestral deleterious alteration) [21]. The BRCA2-8765delAG mutation was firstly described in breast cancer families from French-Canadian and Jewish-Yemenite populations; however, the families from French Canadian and Jewish-Yemenite populations were demonstrated to present with distinct genetic assets at the BRCA2 locus, arguing thus against a common origin of this mutation among such different populations (it seems to be conducted to the high propensity to deletion error in this part of the BRCA2 gene, within a so-called hot-spot mutational region) [22] (**Table 2**).

Few BRCA functional mutations account for BRCA-associated cancers among homogenous populations such as Sardinia (a single BRCA2 founder mutation), French-Canadian population (French colonization of the province of Quebec, five recurrent mutations of which one is common with Sardinia BOC family), and Jewish-Yemenite Ashkenazi Jewish families of eastern European ancestry (specific subpopulations; three recurrent founder mutations are known), while more heterogeneous populations tend to display a broad mutation spectrum; founder mutations are specific mutations that appear repeatedly in ethnically defined groups because of a shared common ancestry [23].

The presence of a singleBRCA2 mutation that is extremely rare (in less than 1% of breast cancer cases) is characterized in another isolated population such as Iceland, which explains a substantial proportion of the familial risk of breast cancer in Iceland and accounts for most of the prostate and ovarian cancer observed in families of breast cancer patients [24].

The epidemiological and clinical impact of the BRCA2 founder mutation on cancer in isolated population has been extensively studied, particularly with regard to significantly higher risk of BOC. The mutations fall into cluster region of BRCA-gene and can be associated with significantly higher risk of breast and ovarian cancer in female population and prostate cancer in males.

Women carrying ascertained pathogenic mutations have a higher lifetime risk of the disease. It's estimated that 55–65% of women with a germinal mutation in BRCA1 will develop breast cancer before age 70. In our series, median age of first diagnosis of breast cancer was 42.5 years (range 27 ± 50); the median value increases significantly up to 57 years (range 39 ± 83) in ovarian cancer cases. Approximately 45% of women with a BRCA2 mutation will develop breast cancer by age 70.

BRCA2 mutation carrier patients with a family history of breast cancer have early median onset of 44 years (range 27 ± 54). The increase of median value is even more significant in ovarian cancer patients selected at any age: 59 years (range 48 ± 77).

Cancers related to a BRCA1 mutation are also more likely to be triple-negative breast cancer, which can be more aggressive and difficult to treat. Triple-negative

Gene	Transcript	Coding	Protein	Function	dbSNP	Clinical Significance	Enigma
BRCA1	NM_007294.3	c.1519 A > T	p.Arg507 Ter	Non sense	rs397508880	Pathogenic	Yes
BRCA1	NM_007294.3	c.1513 A > T	p.Lys505 Ter	Non sense	rs397508877	Pathogenic	Yes
BRCA1	NM_007294.3	c.799 dupT	p.Ser267 fs	Frame shift deletion	rs80357724	Pathogenic	Yes
BRCA1	NM_007294.3	c.981_982 del	p.Cys328 fs	Frame shift deletion	rs80357772	Pathogenic	No*
BRCA1	NM_007294.3	c.1380 dupA	p.F461Ifs	Frame shift deletion	rs80357714	Pathogenic	Yes
BRCA1	NM_007294.3	c.1953 delG	Lys654 Ser	Frame shift deletion	rs80357522	Pathogenic	Yes
BRCA1	NM_007294.3	c.190 T > C	p.Cys64 Arg	Missense	rs80357064	Pathogenic	Yes
BRCA2	NM_000059.3	c.8533_8534 AG	p.Glu2846fs	Frame shift deletion	rs80359714	Pathogenic	Yes
BRCA2	NM_000059.3	c.7683_7684 del	p.Gln2561fs	Frame shift deletion	rs766251541	Pathogenic	Yes
BRCA2	NM_000059.3	c.815 A > T	p.Asn272 Ile	Missense	rs1555067189	Pathogenic	Yes
BRCA2	NM_000059.3	c.6037 A > T	p.Lys2013 Ter	Nonsense	rs80358840	Pathogenic	Yes
BRCA2	NM_000059.3	c.2808_2811delACAA	p.Ala938fs	Frame shift deletion	rs80359351	Pathogenic	Yes

Indicates a variant classified as pathogenic by only ClinVar database and not provided by Enigma.

Table 2.
Variants detected by NGS BRCA panel. Classification criteria were according to the enigma 2015 database.

breast cancer has been classified as a breast cancer subgroup with lack of ER, PR, and HER2 expression and accounts for 15 to 20% of breast cancer cases. Despite a notably favorable rate of response to chemotherapy, triple-negative patients present with a higher risk of relapse and a relatively poor outcome [25].

3. BRCA-related treatments

For breast cancer, treatment options depend on the stage of disease and other factors such as tumor size, results of specific pathology tests (hormone receptors, HER2 receptors, grade of the cells, and proliferation rate of the cells), family history or other risk factors associated with a predisposition for developing breast or ovarian cancer, and age.

Most women with ductal carcinoma in situ (DCIS), a noninvasive breast cancer, have breast-conserving surgery, also known as lumpectomy followed by radiation therapy [26]. Chemotherapy before surgery in women with large stage II or IIIA breast tumors is neo-adjuvant therapy to make possible that breast-conserving surgery. Moreover, after surgery, adjuvant therapy and radiation treatment lower the chance of breast cancer returning [27].

The presence of positive hormone receptor tumor cells is called estrogen receptor-positive (ER-positive) breast cancer; standard hormone therapy (tamoxifen) is based on drug administration that blocks the action of estrogen or prevents it from binding to the estrogen receptor [28]. Among women whose tumors do not express the estrogen receptor (ER-negative breast cancer) and are positive for progesterone receptor (PR), tamoxifen has no effect on recurrence [29].

Herceptin (trastuzumab) can be used to treat HER2-positive breast cancer that is either early-stage or advanced stage/metastatic [30]; it is a humanized monoclonal antibody, specifically used in breast carcinomas in which the HER2/neu transmembrane protein is overexpressed [31]. Herceptin is currently approved to treat metastatic HER2-positive breast cancer to stop the cancer from growing; to treat earlier stages of HER2-positive breast cancer, either as part of a regimen with chemotherapy or alone after a chemotherapy regimen that includes an anthracycline; and to reduce the risk of the breast cancer coming back (recurrence) [32], in combination with pertuzumab and docetaxel before surgery to treat HER2-positive, early-stage (the cancer must be larger than 2 cm or cancer must be in the lymph nodes), inflammatory, or locally advanced-stage breast cancer with a high risk of metastasizing or becoming fatal [33]. Moreover, adjuvant treatment (after surgery) with the combination of pertuzumab, trastuzumab, and chemotherapy significantly reduces the risk of recurrence of breast cancer or death in women with early-stage cancer HER2-positive compared to the therapeutic standard consisting of trastuzumab and chemotherapy [34].

Patients with advanced diagnosis of ovarian cancer are expected to relapse within 3 years, after standard treatment with surgery and chemotherapy (carboplatin-Taxol) [35]. Platinum-based therapy continues to be the principal regimen used to treat ovarian tumors that recur at least 6 months after prior therapy [36].

Carboplatin monotherapy is very convenient to administer, is well tolerated, and produces relatively high response rates (RRs). However, the response usually lasts for only a few months, and with each subsequent course of therapy, the treatment-free interval usually becomes shorter until the tumor is declared 'platinum resistant.' Several studies have combined platinum-based drugs with other agents. Combinations increase the tumor RR and extend the progression-free survival (PFS) [37, 38].

Targeted therapy of 'platinum-sensitive' recurrent OC is conducted in patients at different stages of the treatment pathway. Two classes of drug are being extensively explored in the 'platinum-sensitive' group. These are inhibitors of angiogenesis, an important driver of tumor growth, with a humanized monoclonal antibody, bevacizumab, directed against circulating vascular endothelial growth factor (VEGF) A, an important ligand that binds to the VEGF receptor (VEGFR), stimulating angiogenesis and poly-ADP ribose polymerase (PARP) inhibitors that are active in patients with BRCA gene mutations, and those deficient in the repair of DNA damage through homologous recombination [39, 40].

A germline mutation in one BRCA1 or BRCA2 (gBRCAm) allele is associated with a high risk of the development of a number of cancers, including breast, ovarian, and prostate cancer [41, 42]. Heterozygous BRCA mutations determine loss of function of the remaining wild-type allele, resulting in deficient homologous-recombination DNA repair, which causes genetic aberrations that drive carcinogenesis; the inactivation of the wild-type allele in the tumor is thought to be an obligate step in this process [43, 44].

This tumor-specific defect can be exploited by using PARP inhibitors (e.g., olaparib) to induce selective tumor cytotoxicity, sparing normal cells. Poly(ADP-ribose) polymerase (PARP) is an enzyme involved in base excision repair mechanisms, enabling the adjustment of DNA single-strand breaks repair [45]. Different Parp inhibitors were approved by US FDA: olaparib was approved for use in women with deleterious germline BRCA mutated advanced ovarian cancer and deleterious gBRCAm HER2-negative metastatic breast cancer, while rucaparib was approved for use in women with germline and/or somatic BRCA mutation in advanced ovarian cancer. Several additional Parp inhibitors are in late-phase clinical trials [46].

PARP inhibition in mutated tumor cells with deficient homologous-recombination repair generates unrepaired DNA single-strand breaks that are likely to cause the accumulation of DNA double-strand breaks and collapsed replication forks [47, 48]. Contrariwise, the normal tissue cells that are heterozygous for BRCA mutations and that therefore retain homologous-recombination function have a sensitivity to PARP inhibitors similar to that of wild-type cells, predicting a high therapeutic effect for PARP inhibition in BRCA carriers [49, 50].

The benefits of olaparib (as inhibitor of poly-adenosine diphosphate ribose polymerase) are already widely known in disease relapses. The SOLO-1 study, a double-blind, randomized, prospective phase 3 trial, went to explore for the first time the effects of olaparib as a maintenance therapy, immediately after surgery and chemotherapy, in the newly diagnosed tumor forms, advanced (phase III-IV), BRCA mutated, with a partial or complete clinical response after chemotherapy. Results of the study are encouraging: after a median follow-up of 41 months, the risk of disease progression and/or mortality was 70% lower in patients treated with olaparib than in the control group [51].

4. Conclusions

Genetic testing for breast and ovarian cancer has clinical importance for identification of potentially affected families and for cancer prevention. Approximately, only 5–10% of breast and ovarian cancer are familiar.

Sardinia population shows genetic peculiarity due to geographical isolation and strong genetic drift. The geographical distribution of BRCA1–2 mutations is related to three specific large areas of Sardinia, reflecting its ancient history: the Northern area, linguistically different from the rest of the island where a BRCA2-8765delAG mutation with founder effect, already displayed in our previously study, is predominant [19]. Considering the incidence of the BRCA2-8765delAG variant among the unselected patients from the Sardinian population, our extensive past screening clearly indicated that such a mutation is recurrent in North Sardinia, confirming its role as founder mutation in this part of the island but absent in South Sardinia [52].

Breast cancer families originating from South Sardinia, where BRCA1 mutations are demonstrated to be much more prevalent, present markedly higher rates of association with ovarian cancer [12].

BRCA2 mutations were notably more recurrent than BRCA1 mutations in breast cancer families from North Sardinia and less than 10% of breast cancer families presented an association with ovarian cancer (at least one affected family member) [17]. Nevertheless, the presence of ovarian cancer was demonstrated to significantly increase the occurrence of BRCA1/2 germline mutations in Sardinian breast cancer families [12, 19].

The incidence and mortality trends of ovarian cancer in North Sardinia remained relatively stable in the last decade with cumulative risk of death from the disease being low. Furthermore, survival of patients with ovarian cancer was relatively good in the area, sanctioning the adequacy of the preventive and clinical measures employed in the management of the disease. As for other malignancies, concurrence of different environmental factors and genetic backgrounds may determine the incidence of ovarian cancer.

4.1 Future perspectives

The identification of pathogenic mutations makes it possible to identify, within familial cases, a subpopulation of individuals who present mutations in BRCA-genes. In this classification, however, individuals in whom deleterious mutations could not be identified are excluded, despite having an important family history. Furthermore, the uncertain variants of two major genes do not explain the cancer susceptibility to germ cells.

The future venue of this study is to extend the analysis to possible minor breast cancer susceptibility genes involved in homologous recombination pathways and in repair mechanisms, thanks to the use of increasingly advanced sequencing technologies that involve the use of multigene cancer panels. Functional study and bioinformatics prediction tools provide a putative clinical significance for the identification of somatic variants of interaction between BRCA1 and DNA repair genes and may contribute to identify a role many genes in cancer development.

Acknowledgements

The authors are always grateful to patients for their cooperation during the various studies. This work was funded by Sardinia Regional Government (Regione Autonoma Sardegna) and Italian Association for Research on Cancer (AIRC).

Conflict of interest

All authors declare the absence of any conflict of interest.

Notes/Thanks/Other declarations

A special thanks goes to Oncologic Units of Sardinia for providing cases and clinical information for the study.

Author details

Grazia Palomba[1*], Giuseppe Palmieri[2], Antonio Cossu[3], Panagiotis Paliogiannis[4] and Maria Cristina Sini[1]

1 Institute of Biomolecular Chemistry, National Research Council (CNR), Sassari, Italy

2 Institute of Genetic and Biomedical Research, National Research Council (CNR), Sassari, Italy

3 Anatomia Patologica, Azienda Ospedaliero Universitaria (AOU), Sassari, Italy

4 Unit of Experimental Pathology and Oncology, Department of Medical Surgical and Experimental Sciences, University of Sassari, Sassari, Italy

*Address all correspondence to: graziap68@yahoo.it

References

[1] International Agency for Research on Cancer. Cancer Incidence, Mortality Worldwide. France, GLOBOCAN: IARC Press; 2008. Available from: http://globocan.iarc.fr

[2] Ferlaya J, Steliarova-Fouchera E, Lortet-Tieulent J, et al. Cancer incidence and mortality patterns in Europe: Estimates for 40 countries in 2012. European Journal of Cancer. 2013;**49**(6):1374-1402. DOI: 10.1016/j.ejca.2012.12.027

[3] Easton DF, Bishop DT, Ford D, Crockford GP. Genetic linkage analysis in familial breast and ovarian cancer: Results from 214 families. The breast cancer linkage consortium. American Journal of Human Genetics. 1993;**52**:678-701

[4] Easton D. Breast cancer genes – What are the real risks? Nature Genetics. 1997;**16**:210-211. DOI: 10.1038/ng0797-210

[5] Chun J, Buechelmaier ES, Powell SN. Rad51 Paralog complexes BCDX2 and CX3 act at different stages in the BRCA1-BRCA2-dependent homologous recombination pathway. Molecular and Cellular Biology. 2013;**33**(2):387-395. DOI: 10.1128/MCB.00465-12

[6] Sowter MH, Ashworth A. BRCA1 and BRCA2 as ovarian cancer susceptibility genes. Carcinogenesis. 2005;**26**(10):1651-1656. DOI: 10.1093/carcin/bgi136

[7] Robson ME, Bradbury AR, Arun B, Domchek SM, Ford JM, Hampel HL, et al. American Society of Clinical Oncology policy statement update: Genetic testing for cancer susceptibility. Journal of Clinical Oncology. 2003;**21**:2397-2406. DOI: 10.1200/JCO.2003.03.189

[8] National Comprehensive Cancer Network: NCCN Clinical Practice Guidelines in Oncology. Available from: http://www.nccn.org/professionals/physician_gls/f_guidelines.asp

[9] Raccomandazioni per l'implementazione del test BRCA nelle pazienti con carcinoma ovarico e nei familiari a rischio elevato di neoplasia. AIOM-SIGU-SBIOC-SIAPEC-IAP; 2019. Available from: https://www.aiom.it›wp-content›uploads›2018/11›2019_Raccomandazioni_BRCA_Ovaio.pdf

[10] Budroni M, Cesaraccio R, Pirino D, et al. Cancer incidence in Sassari Province (1998-2002). In: Curado MP, Edwards B, Shin HR, Storm H, Ferlay J, Heanue M, Boyle P, editors. Cancer Incidence in Five Continents. Lyon: IARC Scientific Publications, IARC, IX; 2007

[11] Nedelcu R, Liede A, Aubé J, Finch A, et al. BRCA mutations in Italian breast/ovarian cancer families. European Journal of Human Genetics. 2002;**10**:150-152. DOI: 10.1038/sj.ejhg.5200755

[12] Palmieri G, Palomba G, Cossu A, et al. BRCA1 and BRCA2 germline mutations in Sardinian breast cancer families and their implications for genetic counseling. Annals of Oncology. 2002;**13**:1899-1907. DOI: 10.1093/annonc/mdf326

[13] Palomba G, Pisano M, Cossu A, Budroni M, Dedola MF, Farris A, et al. Spectrum and prevalence of BRCA1 and BRCA2 germline mutations in Sardinian breast cancer patients through a hospital-based screening. Cancer. 2005;**104**:1172. DOI: 10.1186/1471-2407-9-245

[14] Palomba G, Loi A, Porcu E, et al. Genome-wide association study of susceptibility loci for breast cancer in Sardinian population. BMC

Cancer. 2015;**15**:383. DOI: 10.1186/s12885-015-1392-9

[15] I numeri del cancro in Italia, il rapporto Aiom-Airtum. Intermedia Editore; 2019

[16] Risch HA, McLaughlin JR, Cole DEC, et al. Prevalence and penetrance of germline BRCA1 and BRCA2 mutations in a population series of 649 women with ovariancancer. American Journal of Human Genetics. 2001;**68**:700. DOI: 10.1086/318787

[17] King MC, Marks JH, Mandell JB. Breast and ovarian cancer risks due to inherited mutations in BRCA1 and BRCA2. Science. 2003;**302**:643. DOI: 10.1126/science.1088759

[18] Antoniou A, Pharoah PD, Narod S, Risch HA, Eyfjord JE, et al. Average risks of breast and ovarian cancer associated with BRCA1 or BRCA2 mutations detected in case series unselected for family history: A combined analysis of 22 studies. American Journal of Human Genetics. 2003;**72**:1117. DOI: 10.1086/375033

[19] Palomba G, Loi A, Uras A, et al. A role of BRCA1 and BRCA2germline mutations in breast cancer susceptibility within Sardinian population. BMC Cancer. 2009;**9**:245. DOI: 10.1186/1471-2407-9-245

[20] AIRTUM. Associazione Italiana Registri Tumori. Available from: https://www.registri-tumori.it

[21] Lerer I, Wang T, Peretz T, Sagi M, et al. The 8765delAG mutation in BRCA2 is common among Jews of Yemenite extraction. American Journal of Human Genetics. 1998;**63**:272-274. DOI: 10.1086/301924

[22] Palomba G, Cossu A, Friedman E, et al. Origin and distribution of the BRCA2-8765delAG mutation in breast cancer. BMC Cancer. 2007;7:132. DOI: 10.1186/1471-2407-7-132

[23] Tonin PN, Mes-Masson AM, Futreal PA, et al. Founder BRCA1 and BRCA2 Mutations in French Canadian breast and ovarian cancer families. American Journal of Human Genetics. 1998;**63**(5):1341-1351. DOI: 10.1086/302099

[24] Rafnara T, Benediktsdottir KR, Eldon BJ. BRCA2, but not BRCA1, mutations account for familial ovarian cancer in Iceland: A population-based study. European Journal of Cancer. 2004;**40**(18):2788-2793. DOI: 10.1016/j.ejca.2004.09.008

[25] Foulkes WD, Smith IE, Reis-Filho JS. Triple-negative breast cancer. The New England Journal of Medicine. 2010;**363**:1938-1948. DOI: 10.1056/NEJMra1001389

[26] Julien JP, Bijke N, Fentiman IS, et al. Radiotherapy in breast-conserving treatment for ductal carcinoma in situ: First results of the EORTC randomised phase III trial 10853. The Lancet. 2000;**355**(9203):528-533. DOI: 10.1016/S0140-6736(99)06341-2

[27] Miller E, Lee HJ, Lulla A, Hernandez L, et al. Current treatment of early breast cancer: Adjuvant and neoadjuvant therapy. F1000Research. 2014;**3**:198. DOI: 10.12688/f1000research.4340

[28] Lumachi F, Brunello A, Maruzzo M, et al. Treatment of estrogen receptor-positive breast cancer. Current Medicinal Chemistry. 2013;**20**(5):596-604. DOI: 10.2174/092986713804999303

[29] Paik S, Shak S, Tang G, et al. A multigene assay to predict recurrence of Tamoxifen-treated, node-negative breast cancer. The New England Journal

of Medicine. 2004;**351**:2817-2826. DOI: 10.1056/NEJMoa041588

[30] Vogel CL, Cobleigh MA, Tripathy D, et al. Efficacy and safety of Trastuzumab as a single agent in first-line treatment ofHER2-overexpressing metastatic breast cancer. Journal of Clinical Oncology. 2002;**20**(3):719-726. DOI: 10.1200/JCO.2002.20.3.719

[31] Baselga J. Clinical trials of Herceptin® (trastuzumab). European Journal of Cancer. 2001;**37**(1):18-24. DOI: 10.1016/S0959-8049(00)00404-4

[32] Kordestani LA, Wedam S, Zhang L, et al. First FDA approval of Neoadjuvant therapy for breast cancer: Pertuzumab for the treatment of patients with HER2-positive breast cancer. Clinical Cancer Research. 2014;**20**(21):5359-5364. DOI: 10.1158/1078-0432.CCR-14-1268

[33] Von Minckwitz G, Procter M, De Azambuja E, et al. Adjuvant pertuzumab and trastuzumab in early HER2-positive breast cancer. The New England Journal of Medicine. 2017;**377**:122-131. DOI: 10.1056/NEJMoa1703643

[34] Schneeweiss A, Chia S, Hickish T, Harvey V, et al. Pertuzumab plus trastuzumab in combination with standard neoadjuvant anthracycline-containing and anthracycline-free chemotherapy regimens in patients with HER2-positive early breast cancer: A randomized phase II cardiac safety study. Annals of Oncology. 2013;**24**(9):2278-2284. DOI: 10.1093/annonc/mdt182

[35] Bookman MA, Brady MF, McGuire WP, et al. Evaluation of new platinum-based treatment regimens in advanced-stage ovarian cancer: A phase III trial of the gynecologic cancer InterGroup. Journal of Clinical Oncology. 2009;**27**(9):1419-1425. DOI: 10.1200/JCO.2008.19.1684

[36] Markman M, Rothman R, Hakes T, Reichman B, et al. Second-line platinum therapy in patients with ovarian cancer previously treated with cisplatin. Journal of Clinical Oncology. 1991;**9**:389-393. DOI: 10.1200/JCO.1991.9.3.389

[37] Parmar M, Ledermann J, Colombo N, Du Bois A, et al. Paclitaxel plus platinum-based chemotherapy versus conventional platinum-based chemotherapy in women with relapsed ovarian cancer: The ICON4/AGO-OVAR-2.2 trial. Lancet. 2003;**361**:2099-2106. DOI: 10.1016/s0140-6736(03)13718-x

[38] Pujade-Lauraine E, Wagner U, Aavall-Lundqvist E, et al. Pegylated liposomal doxorubicin and carboplatin compared with paclitaxel and carboplatin for patients with platinum-sensitive ovarian cancer in late relapse. Journal of Clinical Oncology. 2010;**28**:3323-3329. DOI: 10.1200/JCO.2009.25.7519

[39] Luvero D, Milani A, Ledermann JA. Treatment options in recurrent ovarian cancer: Latest evidence and clinical potential. Therapeutic Advances in Medical Oncology. 2014;**6**(5):229-239. DOI: 10.1177/1758834014544121

[40] Yap T, Sandhu S, Carden C, De Bono J. Poly(ADP-ribose) polymerase (PARP) inhibitors: Exploiting a synthetic lethal strategy in the clinic. CA: A Cancer Journal for Clinicians. 2011;**61**:31-49. DOI: 10.3322/caac.20095

[41] Wooster R, Weber BL. Breast and ovarian cancer. The New England Journal of Medicine. 2003;**348**:2339-2347. DOI: 10.1056/NEJMra012284

[42] Stratton JF, Gayther SA, Russell P, et al. Contribution of BRCA1 mutations to ovarian cancer. The New England Journal of Medicine.

1997;**336**:1125-1130. DOI: 10.1056/NEJM199704173361602

[43] Maxwell KN, Wubbenhorst B, Wenz BM, Sloover D, et al. BRCA locus-specific loss of heterozygosity in germline BRCA1 and BRCA2 carriers. Nature Communications. 2017;**8**:319. DOI: 10.1038/s41467-017-00388-9

[44] Prakash R, Zhang Y, Feng W, Jasin M. Homologous recombination and human health: The roles of BRCA1, BRCA2, and associated proteins. Cold Spring Harbor Perspectives in Biology. 2015;7(4):a016600. DOI: 10.1101/cshperspect.a016600

[45] Brown JS, O'Carrigan B, et al. Targeting DNA repair in cancer: Beyond PARP inhibitors. Cancer Discovery. 2017;7(1):20-37. DOI: 10.1158/2159-8290

[46] Kamel D, Gray C, Walia JS, Kumar V. PARP inhibitor drugs in the treatment of breast, ovarian, prostate and pancreatic cancers: An update of clinical trials. Current Drug Targets. 2018;**19**(1):21-37(17). DOI: 10.2174/1389450118666170711151518

[47] Farmer H, McCabe N, Lord CJ, et al. Targeting the DNA repair defect in BRCA mutant cells as a therapeutic strategy. Nature. 2005;**434**:917-921. DOI: 10.1038/nature03445

[48] Ashworth A. A synthetic lethal therapeutic approach: Poly(ADP) ribose polymerase inhibitors for the treatment of cancers deficient in DNA double-strand break repair. Journal of Clinical Oncology. 2008;**26**:3785-3790. DOI: 10.1200/JCO.2008.16.0812

[49] Tutt AN, Lord CJ, McCabe N, et al. Exploiting the DNA repair defect in BRCA mutant cells in the design of new therapeutic strategies for cancer. Cold Spring Harbor Symposia on Quantitative Biology. 2005;**70**:139-148. DOI: 10.1101/sqb.2005.70.012

[50] Brody LC. Treating cancer by targeting a weakness. The New England Journal of Medicine. 2005;**353**:949-950. DOI: 10.1056/NEJMcibr052331

[51] Moore K, Colombo N, Scambia G, et al. Maintenance Olaparib in patients with newly diagnosed advanced ovarian cancer. The New England Journal of Medicine. 2018;**379**(26):2495-2505. DOI: 10.1056/NEJMoa1810858

[52] Pisano M, Cossu A, Persico I, Palmieri G, et al. Identification of a founder BRCA2 mutation in Sardinia. British Journal of Cancer. 2000;**82**:553-559. DOI: 10.1054/bjoc.1999.0963

Chapter 5

Genetic Mutation Carriers: Special Considerations for Their Influence on a Modern Breast Reconstruction Practice

Ashley A. Woodfin and Anuja K. Antony

Abstract

With medical advancement, increasing numbers of genetic variations and mutations are being uncovered that offer greater insight into which patients have a predisposition for the development of breast cancer. Reasonable management for these patients includes high-risk surveillance, medical prophylaxis, or bilateral prophylactic mastectomy with immediate reconstruction which is becoming increasingly popular. However, this cohort of patients differs from the average breast cancer patient in that they are typically younger and may have distinct reconstructive objectives for their outcomes. This chapter considers this unique and expanding population, as well as their expectations for surgical outcomes both aesthetically and oncologically. We will discuss the evolving role of social media in this population, with patient to patient virtual information sharing and how this may impact patient referrals in a manner diverging from traditional hospital-based patterns. Furthermore, we discuss how practices in which cutting-edge and novel surgical treatments are available, such as pre-pectoral and single stage reconstruction, and that incorporate team collaboration with the surgical oncologist to deliver aesthetically pleasing results with nipple sparing mastectomy and concealed scars may ultimately be attractive to genetic mutation carriers concerned not only with risk reduction but also post-operative aesthetics.

Keywords: bilateral prophylactic mastectomy, genetic mutation carriers, breast reconstruction, referrals, direct to implant reconstruction

1. Introduction

Primed with internet and social media, high risk breast cancer patients today are increasingly aware of potential outcomes, both oncologic and aesthetic. Modern surgeons today are adapting to an era of technology where patients are empowered like never before. Patients are connected through online groups where they can support each other, share information regarding their treatment and discuss management well ahead of their surgical consultation. The era of the "simply grateful" patients has been replaced with an increasingly sophisticated generation of patients who can access information rapidly and network with other individuals facing similar decisions. Patients have the power to investigate, rate and review their physicians and surgeons through online platforms, the results of which can have significant implications for a practitioner.

Considering the relative ease of obtaining information about surgical options coupled with patients' growing self-awareness regarding their own health, the high-risk breast cancer patient population now confronts a myriad of surgical options. Decisions regarding bilateral prophylactic mastectomy (BPM) are being contemplated by high risk mutation carriers who wish to not only elude breast cancer's grasp, but also remain physically attractive, feminine and desirable. In addition, awareness from prominent public figures and known mutation carriers, such as Angelina Jolie, has drawn admirers and critics alike for their decision to undergo BPM and reconstruction in the absence of cancer; surgeons must now adapt to a younger generation of patients with an elevated consciousness. A surgeon today must not only be constantly on top of the literature associated with breast cancer care, they must also evolve their practice to be cognizant that patients now may seek out their surgeons via less traditional methods. Online reviews, Facebook groups and virtual patient to patient interactions, which were once reserved for identifying high quality eating establishments, are now being used to distinguish high quality surgeons from a menu of practitioners. Physicians practicing in today's medical environment can no longer rely solely on traditional methods of establishing credibility such as pedigree, years of practice, and direct physician to physician recommendations. Google searches, medical review sites, online communities and social media can significantly impact a patient's impression of MD integrity and excellence.

The genetic mutation carrier (GMC) female patient seeking risk reduction surgery with reconstruction is unique and we hope to elucidate how a surgeon can navigate their associated unique considerations and enhanced expectations, both aesthetic and oncologic. We will discuss the role of social media for patient-to-patient virtual experience sharing, as well online physician review websites in regard to referral practices [1]. Furthermore, we will clarify what referral practices contributed to our institution's recent surge in the GMC patient population. In addition, we will discuss optimal collaboration between the surgical oncologist and plastic surgeon needed to provide cutting-edge surgical treatment and novel surgical techniques such as prepectoral (above the muscle) and direct to implant (single stage) reconstruction, as well as how these practices may attract future patients.

2. Decisions facing a younger population of breast surgery patients

GMCs are an emerging population of patients with unique characteristics, perspective, and expectations of surgery. Only 1 out of every 400 people in the general population is estimated to be a BRCA1/2 mutation holder, with ~5–10% of breast cancers at all ages being associated with an inherited gene mutation [2]. Currently the BRCA1/2, ATM, CHEK2, PALB2, TP53, PTEN, CH1, STK11, NBN, NF1 mutations all confer increased risk for breast cancer development, warranting the consideration of BPM for risk reduction [3]. Overall, we expect a 12% lifetime risk of breast cancer development in the general population without any risk factors [4]. This risk increases to 45–65% by age 70 in the population of known mutation carriers of BRCA1/2 [2]. BPM has been shown to reduce the risk by roughly 90% in high risk populations [3], with prophylactic mastectomy and immediate reconstruction becoming increasingly more popular [5, 6]. However, not all GMCs choose BPM, some may prefer to elect chemoprophylaxis or high-risk surveillance instead. This decision is often determined by patient factors, with a recent study showing that GMCs choosing BPM over surveillance tend to have a college education, income

>$50,000, a first-degree relative with breast cancer, higher total number of relatives with breast cancer, and a prior pregnancy [7].

Frequently, woman does not receive a GMC status until after they are diagnosed with a cancer, generally at a younger age. Additionally, many are also being found prior to a cancer diagnosis because of a previously diagnosed family member that underwent that genetic work-up. With these avenues to diagnosis as a GMC, these patients are younger than the average breast cancer patient when they first see a surgeon. This younger age often plays a major role in the decisions these patients make regarding risk reduction surgery and reconstruction.

GMCs that elect for BPM and reconstruction tend to have higher aesthetic expectations than those who require the procedure for treatment of active cancer. There are multiple reasons for this, chief among them being that prophylactic surgery is not considered 'life-saving' and that the patients are at a point in life where cosmesis may play a larger factor. The heightened concern for looking 'natural' and 'unoperated' is an ongoing driver for novel surgical treatments when caring for a patient in this cohort.

In addition, unlike a breast cancer patient, GMC patients have the option of choosing when they want to undergo BPM. Certain life factors can greatly influence when a patient decides to ultimately undergo this prophylactic surgery in her lifetime. Large life events such as marriage and having children can be a major concern in this younger population. Additionally, bilateral mastectomies eliminate the possibility of a woman breastfeeding her children, which many women value as an important bonding experience between mother and child. Aspiring mothers considering BPM may not want to sacrifice this opportunity and timing will be an important factor. A GMC patient's decision regarding surgical timing for BPM is completely personal, and ultimately weighs quality of life with the risk of breast cancer development during the delay. Thus, in a patient strongly desiring to breastfeed her children, family planning plays a very important role in timing for BPM.

3. Long term considerations: implant longevity, surveillance

Yet another facet of caring for the younger age breast surgery patient population is regarding the long-term durability of their reconstruction following BPM. Historically, it has been recommended that patients who underwent cosmetic breast augmentation have their implants exchanged approximately every 10 years. This was after a study published in 1995 found that 81% of implants studied at 10 years were found to have been ruptured [8, 9]. However, due to advancements in implant technology resulting in increased stability of silicone implants using cohesive gel cross-linking technology and thicker implant shells, it is suggested that silicone implants today have greater longevity, but still are not considered 'lifetime devices'. A patient can expect her implants to last at least a decade, with a 1% risk of rupture per year [10]. Another source estimates the new cohesive silicone implants to have a lifetime of 25–35 years [11]. Considering that women may be undergoing BPM with immediate reconstruction as early as their second and third decades of life, they would be expected to live another 50 or greater years following this surgery. Over this long of a timespan, a patient's implants may experience significant degradation, even considering new implant technology, with future surgery for replacement being considered by many an eventuality [10, 11].

It is important to remember that implant-based breast reconstruction comes with risk of prosthesis rupture, albeit minimal. Commonly, silicone implant rupture is related to the normal aging of the prosthesis, but can also rarely be caused by forceful blunt trauma [11]. Implant rupture can occur both silently (without symptom development) or symptomatically, and is also classified as being intracapsular or extracapsular in nature. Intracapsular rupture is defined as being contained within the fibrous breast capsule, whereas extracapsular rupture is more concerning and consists of extravasated silicone gel outside of the fibrous capsule into the surrounding tissues and can lead to inflammation and granuloma formation [11]. Extracapsular rupture is a rare occurrence with silicone implants [29], especially considering the high cohesive types used today. At this time, formal recommendations from the FDA include screening for silent rupture in patients with silicone implants using MRI at 3 years following prosthesis placement, and then every 2 years thereafter [12]. However, a recent meeting of the advisory panel to the FDA released recommendations for revision in implant rupture screening guidelines in late March 2019. These updated recommendations consist of MRI screening at 5–6 years post-operatively, and then every 2–3 years thereafter, with ultrasound being an acceptable alternative to MRI for screening in asymptomatic patients [13]. Unfortunately, these amendments are considered just panel recommendations to the FDA at this time, with the notion that they will be formally adopted by the agency in the upcoming months.

Another critical consideration in this patient population is that of continued surveillance following BPM and reconstruction. As discussed earlier, GMC patients need to be educated about the persistent need for surveillance despite prior mastectomy. Patients should understand that although the majority of breast tissue is removed, the small amount left behind can still ultimately allow for cancer development. Traditional surveillance with mammography is not an option following BPM with reconstruction, requiring this responsibility be placed on the patient and her physicians. Bearing this in mind, it is important for these patients to continue to follow with medical practitioners regularly. Furthermore, self-breast examination and awareness is encouraged to monitor for the formation of any new bumps or irregularities, as these could be cancer development from remnant breast tissue.

Considering all the long-term matters discussed above, it is essential for both the surgical oncologist and plastic surgeon to fully discuss these factors with prospective BPM and reconstruction patients. These factors may play important roles in the choice of those extremely adverse to further procedures, and may ultimately influence their decision regarding whether or not prophylactic surgery is the optimal way to manage their GMC status.

4. Prophylactic surgery and high expectations

Reconstructive expectations of breast cancer patients have evolved greatly over the past few decades with quality of life and survivorship becoming a central focus. This is especially true when treating GMCs, putting a greater demand on the surgical collaboration required for successful execution. Today, it is not uncommon for patients to expect their post-surgical breasts to improve their appearance and more closely match their desired size and shape than their pre-surgery breast aesthetic. Ultimately, the GMC patient has a choices regarding surgical timing, type and the decision to pursue surgery or not, so expectations are inherently high.

One reason for this rise may be the downstream effect of popular culture with increasing acceptance for a GMC's surgical choices, normalizing the idea of having a bilateral mastectomy with reconstruction for risk reduction, while also demonstrating the fact that a woman can still be considered desirable and attractive after this surgery. Angelina Jolie, through a series of op-ed pieces written for the New York Times and other media outlets, recounted her personal journey with having the BRCA mutation, the passing of her mother from ovarian cancer, and her surgical choices for BPM and reconstruction. She single-handedly has perhaps most profoundly affected public opinion regarding BPM and amplified awareness for a GMC's breast cancer risk. Today, the modern GMC female interested in BPM expects she will retain her femininity and ability to identify as a beautiful woman post-operatively.

For the modern surgeon, it is important to convey a confident, but realistic depiction of the likely outcomes during the pre-operative consultation. This includes discussion of individual patient factors that can influence the final aesthetic outcome such as BMI, current breast size and ptosis, as well as the possibility of requiring revisional procedures in the future (e.g., fat grafting). Patients with realistic expectations of their reconstructive journey and cosmetic outcomes have been shown more likely to be satisfied with their BPM results. Additionally, it appears that patients who discuss BPM with their partners prior are more likely to be satisfied with intimacy post-operatively [14].

5. Online era: social media and patient influence

Social media plays an ever-expanding role in our lives. There are many online support groups for mutation carriers that easily and immediately connect patients around the world [15]. Within these online groups, and social media in general, now exists a special category of users referred to as 'influencers'. These are users who cultivate a particularly large community of 'followers' with which they share experiences, ideas, products, and influence the general attitudes of those that follow them. It is not uncommon to see an individual sharing their entire experience as a 'mutation carrier,' 'cancer thriver,' or 'cancer survivor' on some form of social media (e.g., Instagram, Facebook, or a blog) [15]. This influence is not confined to the normal events of everyday life, but also extends to health decisions. Since the experiences of one person can be so easily disseminated, the clinical course and opinions of a single patient can disproportionally reverberate throughout the entire community. This process can act as an endorsement for, or dissuasion against, a certain treatment, surgery, or surgeon depending on the level of satisfaction of a single patient. This is particularly important to a surgeon's referral-based practice as the large social media following of certain patients can have greater consequences, both good and bad, to their "business" than seen historically.

Moreover, online review sites for patients to publicly rate their physicians are becoming more and more prevalent. Patients are taking control over who they choose for their care, and this does not exclude surgeons. Many visit these websites prior to committing their care to a certain surgeon, and use the information presented there to help guide their decision. Yet, an important question needs to be addressed: do the ratings on these websites actually correlate with the clinical outcomes achieved by the physicians? Recently this has become an area of intrigue in the surgical community, and over the past few years, a handful of small studies were published exploring the possible correlation between online health ratings of surgeons and their surgeon-specific measurable outcomes. Some of these investigated outcomes include infection rate, re-admission rate, revisional surgery rate, and risk-adjusted mortality rate, in surgeries such as total knee replacements, hernia repairs, and coronary artery bypass grafting. All of these studies failed to find any correlation between a surgeon's online ratings and their measurable outcomes, including those listed above [16–18]. These results seriously undermine the utility of such websites, however are unlikely to be realized by the average health care consumer.

Furthermore, a similar study went one step further to try and identify what positively versus negatively influences a physician's rating by reading and analyzing the written reviews/comments on these websites. In order to accomplish this, the reviews were read by study staff and comments were classified as being either surgeon-dependent factors (competence or likeability) or surgeon-independent factors (office environment, staff, billing, etc.). Interestingly, this study found that comments on surgeon-dependent factors were associated with higher ratings, and furthermore that comments on surgeon-independent factors were associated with lower ratings [19]. This ultimately reinforces the results of the previously discussed studies, that physician ratings are not associated with outcomes, but rather highly influenced by office interactions. However, it does emphasize the importance of a good bedside manner for the surgeon, as well as his office staff, in addition to bringing awareness to the significance of the overall perceived patient experience when rating their physician on these websites—not unlike how a patron would consider their entire culinary dining experience and not just their food to formulate a restaurant review.

6. Our experience: what guides patient referrals

To better understand how the internet and social media affects patient referrals, we reviewed our patient database and identified recent GMCs in the absence of cancer ($n = 10$) that underwent BPM with immediate reconstruction at our institution. GMCs without a current diagnosis of cancer were of interest as they are inherently less pressured to make surgical decisions. Given these patients did not have active cancer, they had the advantage of taking as much time as they needed to research online, look for personal referrals, and read online health grade reviews before making their decision. Theoretically, they also had less tying them to a specific institution given no cancer diagnostic information had to be transferred from one institution to another. Patients' referral patterns were reviewed and, if interested, were asked to complete a telephone survey (70% response rate) regarding their decision to pursue surgery at our institution.

Many stated that they first chose to undergo consultation at our institution because of internal referrals from physicians they already trusted. Most notably the patients stated their referrals tended to come from OB/GYNs when looking a surgical oncologist, and from the surgical oncologist when looking for a plastic surgeon. This emphasizes the importance of a strong collaborative relationship between the two surgeons.

The majority stated that the aspect of utmost importance in confirming their decision was feeling confident and comfortable with their surgeons after meeting them for initial consultations. Many women stated that their interactions with both the surgical oncologist and plastic surgeon were very open and honest, especially in taking the time to answer all the patients' questions. They felt a strong personal connection with their surgeons and the warmth they experienced helped build trust, which comforted them and positively influenced their decision to receive care at our institution.

For many, the internet and social media served as a resource affirming their decision to receive care at our institution. One patient detailed that her surgical oncologist was mentioned favorably in Facebook groups, and plastic surgeon was known to have a great reputation online as well, but noted that this did not primarily drive her decision. Approximately one third of the patients looked at online health reviews and ratings for their surgeons prior to committing care to our institution, and stated again that these served to positively reinforce their decision.

When asked about the most important factor regarding these surgeries, the majority of former patients stated that risk reduction was most important to them, however cosmetic outcomes were found to be almost equally as important. Younger patients appeared more concerned with cosmetic outcomes. In regard to novel surgical techniques attracting patients and influencing their decisions, most stated that the possibility of having single stage, also known as direct to implant (DTI), reconstruction was very appealing to them, and was sought out. Knowing that their plastic surgeon was a specialist in prepectoral DTI reconstruction was important to these women as well. However, not all were candidates for this option at initial consultation, but this fact did not dissuade their ultimate decision.

7. Novel reconstructive techniques: a patient attractor

We believe that in ultimately selecting a plastic surgeon for their breast reconstructive needs, the modern GMC patient not only evaluates outcomes, but also considers surgeons performing state-of-the-art procedures, using the newest technologies and novel techniques, especially when they offer obvious advantages to the patient. This includes pre-pectoral implant placement, as well as single stage (also referred to as direct to implant (DTI)) reconstruction. Though not necessarily actively sought out by all, the possibility of being able to have immediate single stage reconstruction could solidify a patient's decision to receive care with a certain plastic surgeon by offering them the option of a shortened reconstructive course. More recently popularized mastectomy techniques such as the nipple sparring mastectomy (NSM), when oncologically appropriate, are being more actively sought out from oncologic surgeons as well, as they also contribute to more aesthetically pleasing results.

The nipple is generally considered a distinguishing feature of a natural breast. Considering this fact, NSM continues to be increasingly popular with GMCs. In 2018, a review of the American Society of Breast Surgeons (ASBrS) NSM database showed the majority of NSMs as being performed for prophylactic reasons [20]. Furthermore, NSM patients tend to be younger, Caucasian, and have smaller BMIs [21]. Another study showed higher body image scale scores in NSM compared to skin sparring mastectomy (SSM), but the difference was not statistically significant [22]. Other studies have also noted higher psychosocial [23] and sexual wellbeing scores in NSM patients [21].

However, NSM is not without risk; their documented complication rate is low but not insignificant, and includes possible complications to the nipple areolar complex (NAC) such as nipple necrosis and epidermolysis, in addition to infection and mastectomy flap necrosis risk seen in all mastectomies. A recent review of the ASBrS NSM database documented a NAC complication rate of 4.4% [20]. Moreover, there is a statistically significant decrease in the measured sensation of the NAC after NSM when compared to control groups [22]. Unfortunately, this reality of a nipple sparing mastectomy is not always completely understood by patients prior to consultation. Explaining these risks and realities can be more difficult in a patient population that has less tolerance for imperfection because of how it may affect their quality of life. Transparency and informed consent remain critical components to counseling the GMC patient considering BPM.

New techniques in reconstructive surgery are also likely to influence a patient's decision on their surgeon preference. Novel techniques available include the option for prepectoral implant placement, as well as single stage (direct to implant) reconstruction. The availability of these techniques to patients depends on several factors, the first of which being plastic surgeon's experience with the procedures, the patient's current and desired final appearance, as well as mastectomy flap thickness, perfusion and viability.

Two-stage breast reconstruction using tissue expanders placed subpectorally has been the traditional method for immediate breast reconstruction since the 1970s. This technique was developed during a time when mastectomies were more radical, excising more skin in the surgical process. Over time, the progression of mastectomies from modified-radical to skin-sparring, and now nipple-sparing, has increased preservation of the breast envelope and allowed for reconstructive advancements as well. These larger breast envelopes create the option for placing implants at the initial surgery without placing excess tension on the mastectomy flaps. In properly chosen patients, this technique can be employed without an increased risk for complications [24]. Reconstructive surgery performed in two stages has drawbacks that DTI circumvents including the avoidance of multiple episodes of anesthesia [25–28]. Recent studies have also elucidated other possible advantages with DTI, including increased patient satisfaction, reduction in pain, and possible reduction in cost when comparing DTI with two stage reconstruction [25–27]. DTI reconstruction when first introduced capitalized on the safety and advantages of an expanded dual plane pocket using acellular dermal matrix (ADM) as an inferior sling to support implant placement under the pectoralis muscle in a single stage surgery [29, 30]. Despite the perceived benefits, DP DTI reconstructions still retain the same issues created by placing a prosthesis in the subpectoral or dual plane (DP) position, namely animation deformity and pectoralis major origin disruption causing weakened adduction [31].

Prepectoral (PP) implant placement resolved the issue of animation deformity caused by subpectoral placement [31, 32]. However, without routine use of ADM, the subcutaneous or prepectoral techniques were historically fraught with high rates of early capsular contracture [33], flap necrosis, implant loss [34], and concern for worsened aesthetics (e.g., implant visibility, rippling) often requiring additional procedures for revision such as fat grafting. One study compared PP placement with and without the use of ADM, demonstrating significantly lower rates of capsular contracture in the ADM cohort [35]. From our experience, the crucial components necessary for successful PP DTI include initial intraoperative assessment of flap perfusion with sizer in place, followed by the creation of a tight anterior ADM pocket for implant insertion [24]. Use of anterior ADM coverage for implant support and off-loading pressure on the mastectomy flaps prevents the complications traditionally associated with PP [24], while avoiding the disadvantages of DP placement. Despite this, the PP DTI technique has yet to be widely adopted secondary to the lingering concerns over historical complications and the steep learning curve.

Our group performed one of the largest DTI-only comparative study (n = 134) between outcomes of dual plane (DP) DTI and prepectoral (PP) DTI, and showed an overall low complication incidence, with PP DTI complications being slightly less frequent (PP 2% vs. DP 12%, p = 0.07). No implant losses were documented in this study. Furthermore, regarding the concern over increased need for aesthetic revisional procedures in PP patients, no difference was shown in the likelihood of either DP or PP DTI patients to undergo these additional procedures. Last, this study reinforced the positive aesthetic outcomes of PP DTI with a blinded panel scoring PP DTI reconstructions higher than DP DTI in terms of aesthetic outcome [32]. This study effectively corroborated the non-inferiority of PP DTI to DP DTI reconstructive techniques, as well as demonstrated its advantage in better cosmetic outcomes. Because of this, the ability to perform PP DTI could be potentially attractive to patients concerned with aesthetic outcomes when looking for a reconstructive surgeon.

Finally, it should be noted that appropriate patient selection is of utmost importance for successful PP DTI. As explained earlier in this chapter, adequate mastectomy flap perfusion is crucial for employment of this reconstructive technique, and we advocate intra-operative use of fluorescence imaging technology to ensure this. Our group considers active smoking and uncontrolled medical co-morbidities to be absolute contraindications to PP DTI. Whereas, obesity is only considered a relative contraindication and our group has found that the use of oncoplastic reconstructive techniques in conjunction with implant placement has yielded great results. More ideal patients for PP DTI include those desiring results similar to their native breast size [24], though we have found upsizing of the breast to be possible in the compliant envelope.

8. Surgeon collaboration: oncologic and reconstructive considerations

The goal of BPM in GMCs is risk reduction, and in order to achieve this goal, removal of as much breast tissue as possible provides the best oncologic benefit. A mastectomy, while drastically reducing cancer occurrence, does not completely eliminate the possibility of breast cancer development in the future. As tissue removal and oncologic benefit increases, risk benefit must be considered as excessively thin mastectomy flaps incur higher risk for ischemia, complicating reconstructive efforts. Adequate flap vascularity is a critical component to successful breast reconstruction, especially single stage, with thicker flaps conferring less risk of ischemia and flap necrosis [31, 36]. This relationship between removing the maximum amount of breast tissue while retaining flap perfusion are the competing priorities that surgical oncologists and plastic surgeons must navigate effectively together.

Approaching a combined mastectomy/reconstruction patient most importantly requires effective communication between the two surgeons. Additionally, in our institution we employ fluorescence imaging technology in immediate breast reconstruction cases to help quantify perfusion to the flaps [37]. This practice identifies the flaps at risk for ischemia so that the appropriate reconstructive path for each patient can be followed, guiding the decision-making process surrounding whether a patient is more appropriate for one or two stage reconstruction, or delayed reconstruction.

9. Conclusion

Overall, the improved understanding of genetic mutation and risk for breast cancer development has created a special population of breast surgery patients. They have specific priorities that must be considered when it comes to surgical planning, risk tolerance, long term considerations, and both oncologic and aesthetic outcomes. This population's younger age may play a large role in expectations with higher value placed on cosmesis. In response, techniques such as NSM and single stage prepectoral reconstruction are being more commonly used to meet this population's particular demands for excellent outcomes, both oncologic and cosmetic.

Considering our modern online era, we believe that the internet and social media will continue to increasingly affect patient referral patterns. Although online rating and review websites so far have shown no correlation with a surgeon's actual measurable outcomes, it appears as though they continue to be popular information sources for prospective patients and help confirm their decisions on where to receive care. Being mindful of this online presence will be crucial for the successful modern plastic surgery practice, in addition to offering novel surgical techniques to satisfy the expectations of today's patients. However, the traditional practice of upholding a good bedside manner, developing excellent surgeon-patient rapport, and patient trust in their referring physician will continue to be important factors.

Conflict of interest

Dr. Ashley Woodfin has no conflicts of interest to disclose. Dr. Anuja Antony has a consultant agreement with Allergan Medical Inc. She received no compensation or support for this book chapter.

The authors have no financial interest or disclosures to declare related to the content of this manuscript.

Author details

Ashley A. Woodfin[1]* and Anuja K. Antony[2]

1 Department of Surgery, Division of Surgical Oncology, Rush University Medical Center, Chicago, IL, USA

2 Department of Surgery, Division of Plastic and Reconstructive Surgery, Rush University Medical Center, Chicago, IL, USA

*Address all correspondence to: ashley_a_woodfin@rush.edu

References

[1] Woodfin A, Skladman R, Madrigrano A, Antony A. Genetic Mutation Carriers: A growing, evolving, and unique breast surgery population. Submitted

[2] National Cancer Institute. Genetics of breast and gynecologic cancers (PDQ®): Health professional (Version 2018). Available from: https://www.cancer.gov/types/breast/hp/breast-ovarian-genetics-pdq#link/_113_toc [Accessed: 20 January 2019]

[3] National Comprehensive Cancer Network (NCCN). Genetic/Familial High-Risk Assessment: Breast and Ovarian (Version 3.2019). Available from: https://www.nccn.org/professionals/physician_gls/pdf/genetics_screening.pdf [Accessed: 20 January 2019]

[4] Noone AM, Howlader N, Krapcho M, Miller D, Brest A, Yu M, et al., editors. SEER Cancer Statistics Review. Bethesda, MD: National Cancer Institute; 1975-2015. Available from: https://seer.cancer.gov/csr/1975_2015/ [based on November 2017 SEER data submission, posted to the SEER web site, April 2018]

[5] Cemal Y, Albornoz CR, Disa JJ, McCarthy CM, Mehrara BJ, Pusic AL, et al. Paradigm shift in U.S. breast reconstruction: Part 2. The influence of changing mastectomy patterns on reconstructive rate and method. Plastic and Reconstructive Surgery. 2013;**131**(3):320e-326e

[6] Panchal H, Matros E. Current trends in postmastectomy breast reconstruction. Plastic and Reconstructive Surgery. 2017;**140**(5S Advances in Breast Reconstruction):7S-13S

[7] Henry DA, Lee MC, Almanza D, Ahmed KA, Sun W, Boulware DC, Laronga C. Trends in use of bilateral prophylactic mastectomy vs high-risk surveillance in unaffected carriers of inherited breast cancer syndromes in the Inherited Cancer Registry (ICARE). Breast Cancer Research Treatment. Feb 2019;**174**(1):39-45

[8] Robinson OG Jr, Bradley EL, Wilson DS. Analysis of explanted silicone implants: A report of 300 patients. Annals of Plastic Surgery. 1995;**34**(1):1-6; discussion 6-7

[9] Rohrich RJ, Adams WP Jr, Beran SJ, Rathakrishnan R, Griffin J, Robinson JB Jr, et al. An analysis of silicone gel-filled breast implants: Diagnosis and failure rates. Plastic and Reconstructive Surgery. 1998;**102**(7):2304-2308; discussion 2309

[10] Culbertson E. What is the lifespan of breast Implants?. 2017. Available from: https://www.plasticsurgery.org/news/blog/what-is-the-lifespan-of-breast-implants [Accessed: 14 March 2019]

[11] Shikhman R, Moufarrege R. Breast Implant Rupture. StatPearls [Internet]. Treasure Island (FL): StatPearls Publishing; 2019. Available from: http://www-ncbi-nlm-nih-gov.ezproxy.rush.edu/books/NBK459308/ [Accessed: 24 February 2019]

[12] Food and Drug Administration. Silicone Gel-Filled Breast Implants. Updated August 28, 2018. Available from: https://www.fda.gov/medicaldevices/productsandmedicalprocedures/implantsandprosthetics/breastimplants/ucm063871.htm [Accessed: 14 March 2019]

[13] Food and Drug Administration. 24 Hour Summary General and Plastic Surgery Devices Advisory Committee Meeting March 25 & 26,

2019. Available from: https://www.fda.gov/downloads/AdvisoryCommittees/CommitteesMeetingMaterials/MedicalDevices/MedicalDevicesAdvisoryCommittee/GeneralandPlasticSurgeryDevicesPanel/UCM634622.pdf [Accessed: 15 April 2019]

[14] Glassey R, O'Connor M, Ives A, Saunders C, Hardcastle SJ, kConFab Investigators. Influences on satisfaction with reconstructed breasts and intimacy in younger women following bilateral prophylactic mastectomy: A qualitative analysis. International Journal of Behavioral Medicine. 2018;**25**(4):390-398

[15] Stefansdottir V. Experience of social media support group for BRCA carriers. Journal of Genetic Counseling. 2016;**25**(6):1342-1344

[16] Okike K, Peter-Bibb TK, Xie KC, Okike ON. Association between physician online rating and quality of care. Journal of Medical Internet Research. 2016;**18**(12):e324

[17] Trehan SK, Nguyen JT, Marx R, Cross MB, Pan TJ, Daluiski A, et al. Online patient ratings are not correlated with total knee replacement surgeon-specific outcomes. HSS Journal. 2018;**14**(2):177-180. DOI: 10.1007/s11420-017-9600-6. Epub: January 10, 2018

[18] Haskins IN, Krpata DM, Rosen MJ, Perez AJ, Tastaldi L, Butler RS, et al. Online surgeon ratings and outcomes in hernia surgery: An americas hernia society quality collaborative analysis. Journal of the American College of Surgeons. 2017;**225**(5):582-589. DOI: 10.1016/j.jamcollsurg.2017.08.007. Epub August 31, 2017

[19] Donnally CJ 3rd, Roth ES, Li DJ, Maguire JA Jr, McCormick JR, Barker GP, et al. Analysis of internet review site comments for spine surgeons: How office staff, physician likeability, and patient outcome are associated with online evaluations. Spine (Phila Pa 1976). 2018;**43**(24):1725-1730

[20] Mitchell SD, Willey SC, Beitsch P, Feldman S. Evidence based outcomes of the American society of breast surgeons nipple sparing mastectomy registry. Gland Surgery. 2018;7(3):247-257

[21] Romanoff A, Zabor EC, Stempel M, Sacchini V, Pusic A, Morrow M. A comparison of patient-reported outcomes after nipple-sparing mastectomy and conventional mastectomy with reconstruction. Annals of Surgical Oncology. 2018;**25**(10):2909-2916

[22] Van Verschuer VM, Mureau MA, Gopie JP, Vos EL, Verhoef C, Menke-Pluijmers MB, et al. Patient satisfaction and nipple-areola sensitivity after bilateral prophylactic mastectomy and immediate implant breast reconstruction in a high breast cancer risk population: Nipple-sparing mastectomy versus skin-sparing mastectomy. Annals of Plastic Surgery. 2016;**77**(2):145-152

[23] Razdan SN, Patel V, Jewell S, McCarthy CM. Quality of life among patients after bilateral prophylactic mastectomy: A systematic review of patient-reported outcomes. Quality of Life Research. 2016;**25**(6):1409-1421

[24] Antony AK, Robinson EC. An Algorithmic Approach to Prepectoral Direct-to-Implant Breast Reconstruction: Version 2.0. Plastic and Reconstructive Surgery. May 2019;**143**(5):1311-1319

[25] Susarla SM, Ganske I, Helliwell L, Morris D, Eriksson E, Chun YS. Comparison of clinical outcomes and patient satisfaction in immediate single-stage versus two-stage implant-based breast reconstruction.

Plastic and Reconstructive Surgery. 2015;**135**(1):1e-8e

[26] Krishnan NM, Fischer JP, Basta MN, Nahabedian MYI. Direct-to-implant breast reconstruction cost effective? A cost utility analysis of prosthetic breast reconstruction. Plastic and Reconstructive Surgery. 2015;**136** (4 Suppl):110-111

[27] Roostaeian J, Sanchez I, Vardanian A, Herrera F, Galanis C, Da Lio A, et al. Comparison of immediate implant placement versus the staged tissue expander technique in breast reconstruction. Plastic and Reconstructive Surgery. 2012;**129**(6):909e-918e

[28] Glasberg SB. The economics of prepectoral breast reconstruction. Plastic and Reconstructive Surgery. 2017;**140**(6S Prepectoral Breast Reconstruction):49S-52S

[29] Salzberg CA. Nonexpansive immediate breast reconstruction using human acellular tissue matrix graft (AlloDerm). Annals of Plastic Surgery. 2006;**57**(1):1-5

[30] Colwell AS, Damjanovic B, Zahedi B, Medford Davis L, Hertl C, Austen WG. Retrospective review of 331 consecutive immediate single-stage implant reconstructions with acellular dermal matrix: Indications, complications, trends, and costs. Plastic and Reconstructive Surgery. 2011;**128**(6):1170-1178

[31] Jones G, Yoo A, King V, Jao B, Wang H, Rammos C, et al. Prepectoral immediate direct-to-implant breast reconstruction with anterior AlloDerm coverage. Plastic and Reconstructive Surgery. 2017;**140**(6S Prepectoral Breast Reconstruction):31S-38S

[32] Antony AK, Poirier J, Madrigrano A, Kopkash KA, Robinson EC. Evolution of the Surgical Technique for "Breast in a Day" Direct-to-Implant Breast Reconstruction: Transitioning from Dual-Plane to Prepectoral Implant Placement. Plastic and Reconstructive Surgery. Jun 2019;**143**(6):1547-1556

[33] Hammond DC, Schmitt WP, O'Connor EA. Treatment of breast animation deformity in implant-based reconstruction with pocket change to the subcutaneous position. Plastic and Reconstructive Surgery. 2015;**135**(6):1540-1544

[34] Snyderman RK, Guthrie RH. Reconstruction of the female breast following radical mastectomy. Plastic and Reconstructive Surgery. 1971;**47**(6):565-567

[35] Vardanian AJ, Clayton JL, Roostaeian J, Shirvanian V, Da Lio A, Lipa JE, et al. Comparison of implant-based immediate breast reconstruction with and without acellular dermal matrix. Plastic and Reconstructive Surgery. 2011;**128**(5):403e-410e

[36] Qureshi AA, Broderick KP, Belz J, Funk S, Reaven N, Brandt KE, et al. Uneventful versus successful reconstruction and outcome pathways in implant-based breast reconstruction with acellular dermal matrices. Plastic and Reconstructive Surgery. 2016;**138**(2):173e-183e

[37] Munabi NC, Olorunnipa OB, Goltsman D, Rohde CH, Ascherman JA. The ability of intra-operative perfusion mapping with laser-assisted indocyanine green angiography to predict mastectomy flap necrosis in breast reconstruction: A prospective trial. Journal of Plastic, Reconstructive & Aesthetic Surgery. 2014;**67**(4):449-455

Section 2

Breast Conservative Surgery: Oncoplasties

Chapter 6

Oncoplastic Surgery in Breast Cancer

Atallah David, Moubarak Malak and Abdallah Abdallah

Abstract

Oncoplastic surgery is an emerging approach which combines breast-conserving surgery and plastic surgery techniques. It aims to provide wider volume resection with oncologically clear margins and at the same time to maintain the breast shape and optimize cosmetic outcomes. Inspired from esthetic breast surgery techniques, oncoplasty consists of breast volume displacement to fill the defect of large resections and optimize the cosmetic outcomes without interfering with the oncoplastic safety. In this chapter, the concept, indications, and principles of oncoplastic techniques used in conservative breast surgeries will be exposed. A photo-based atlas for oncoplastic incisions will concern seven cases starting with the preoperative planning and marking and ending up with the long-term postoperative outcomes.

Keywords: breast cancer, oncoplasty, oncological safety, cosmetic outcome

1. Introduction

During the last century, breast surgery has witnessed a tremendous evolution leading to radical changes in surgical concepts and standards. In 1894, William S. Halsted published the first results of the known "Halsted radical mastectomy" which consisted of en bloc resection of all suspected tissues including all breast tissue, axillary lymph nodes, and both pectoral muscles [1]. This technique lasted for more than 50 years until Patey and Dyson have introduced the modified radical mastectomy with sparing of the pectoralis muscles [2]. Later in the 1970s with the introduction of the radiotherapy in the management of breast cancer, we started to abandon the "fits all" mastectomy approach as we demonstrated the equivalency of breast-conserving surgery when combined to radiotherapy in comparison to mastectomy. With the comparable survival and recurrence rates between the two approaches published by the Milan trials and the National Surgical Adjuvant Breast and Bowel Project (NSABP) B-04 trial, we entered a new era in the breast cancer management and shifted the paradigm away from the psychological burden that was associated with the mastectomy [3, 4]. Gradually the breast-conserving surgery combined with radiotherapy has become the preferred approach in the case of early breast cancer cases however with high rates of poor cosmetic outcomes (30–40%) and residual deformities, especially when larger volume excision is needed. The failure of classical breast-conserving surgery

IntechOpen

techniques has anticipated the development of new approaches to improve cosmetic outcomes as well as patient satisfaction. From this ideal, the oncoplastic surgery was born in the last two decades [5].

2. Definition and concept

Oncoplastic surgery is a new approach that combines surgical oncological principles with plastic surgical techniques. It aims to provide wide tumor excision with an immediate reshaping of the remaining breast tissue using many forms of remodeling techniques. The goal of oncoplastic surgery is to completely remove the lesion with clear margins and with good to excellent cosmetic result in one definitive procedure [6]. This novel technique does not compromise the oncological safety. At the contrary, it proves good oncological efficacy in terms of margin status and recurrence in comparison to traditional breast-conserving surgery techniques. This could be related to the large breast volume excision and consequently safe margins that this technique provides [7–10]. It is worthy to note that the surgeon can perform this approach with sentinel lymph node biopsy or axillary lymph node dissection.

3. Principle

Before deciding if a patient is eligible to undergo an oncoplastic surgery, we need to consider three factors: excision volume, tumor location, and glandular density [11].

First of all, excision volume is the most predictive factor for poor outcomes. It was suggested that excision of >20% of breast tissue could impair the breast shape and lead to a poor cosmetic outcome [12, 13]. With oncoplastic techniques, the surgeon can remove an average of 200 g up to 1000 g and without interfering with the natural breast shape [14]. A remodeling of the adjacent remaining breast tissue enables the surgeon to fill the defect created by the tumor resection. A preoperative assessment of the breast volume and tumor size as well as a proper evaluation of the imaging findings guides the surgeon in his operative decision.

Second, the tumor location plays an essential role in guiding the incision type and the size of volume excision. For example, correcting a defect after removing a tumor from the upper outer quadrant is easier in comparison to a defect in the upper inner quadrant where less breast tissue is available to be mobilized [11].

Third, the breast density guides the extent of breast undermining and reshaping. A breast with high fat composition limits the tissue manipulation and mobilization and may expose to higher rates of complications especially fat necrosis. A preoperative mammographic evaluation aids in the breast density assessment and helps the surgeon in his operative choice [11].

Additional factors to be considered are:

- The fat content in the axillary area in the case of resection in the outer quadrants
- The size of the breast and its implication on the extent of volume excision
- The grade of ptosis

- The associated clinical conditions, especially smoking, uncontrolled diabetes, or older age that may interfere with the healing process and lead to higher complications rates [15]

4. Preoperative planning

The success of an oncoplastic procedure starts with a good and reasonable preoperative planning. The first issue to be considered is the estimated volume of the tumor relative to the overall breast [15]. Imaging modalities play an important role in the evaluation of the local extent of disease in patients with breast cancer.

Performing a magnetic resonance imaging (MRI) preoperatively helps the surgeon in assessing the extent of disease especially in the case of dense breast tissue. The sensitivity and specificity of MRI are 93–100% and 26–91%, respectively [16–18]. MRI also helps to identify lesions on the contralateral side. Besides, it is useful for the detection of multifocal or multicentric lesions and consequently may alter the surgical management [19]. In a meta-analysis, the authors found that 8.1% of patients were converted from breast-conserving therapy to mastectomy and 11.3% of patients were converted from breast-conserving therapy to more extensive surgery after performing an MRI [20]. Another benefit is that MRI enables the surgeon to assess the amount of fat and dense breast tissue. The surgeon must reconsider both the incision type and the need for mobilization when planning the operation in the case of mostly fatty breasts due to the increased rate of fat necrosis in this type of breasts when manipulated too much.

MRI alone is not sufficient for decision-making and should be combined with mammography. MRI in addition to mammography is an accurate tool to determine the suitability for a breast-conserving surgery. Although MRI predicts the possibility of conservative treatment, this can be improved with the addition of mammography which may increase the extent of the disease compared to that seen on MRI due to the visualization of microcalcifications [21]. Moreover, digital breast tomosynthesis (DBT) has emerged recently as a novel approach permitting to reduce the obscuring effect of overlying breast tissue and to overcome the limitations of the regular mammogram [22–24]. Also integrating the tomosynthesis in the preoperative work-up may increase the diagnostic accuracy of mammographic lesion evaluation and improve the breast cancer staging significantly in patients with dense breasts compared to conventional mammography alone [25, 26].

A mammogram is always complemented with ultrasound examination to localize the mammographic and tomographic lesions. Ultrasound-guided biopsies are needed to confirm the diagnosis as well as to evaluate the axillary lymph node status. Suspicious lymph nodes are evaluated with needle biopsy [6]. Also, wire localization of the tumors is mostly done under ultrasound guidance preoperatively. Sometimes, multiple wires are needed to guide the surgeon in the extent of the resection [27].

Preoperative planning also requires the case presentation in the tumor board where a multidisciplinary team is involved in the decision-making. Oncologic surgeon, radiologist, pathologist, oncologist, radiation oncologist, and others may be included [6]. For a better outcome, the patient can also be implicated in the operative decision.

5. Techniques

Many techniques of oncoplastic incisions were described in the literature. It is not a one technique fits all. In every case, the surgeon needs to take into consideration the tumor size, the volume of the breast, the grade of ptosis, the age of the patients, and other factors without compromising the oncologic safety. Many techniques may be applicable for every tumor location. An experienced surgeon in oncoplastic surgery will be able to decide which technique will provide better oncological as well as cosmetic outcomes. We will cite the most commonly used techniques, and then we will expose photos of the markings as well as postoperative outcomes of seven cases.

We need to distinguish between two types of oncoplastic techniques:

1. Reconstruction of the breast from local breast tissue which may include:

    a. The rotation techniques (rotational/advancement flap) (case 1, 2 and 4)

    b. B-plasty

    c. Tumor-adapted reduction mammoplasty: for lower quadrant lesions, also in the case of severe ptosis (case 3)

    d. Central quadrantectomy

    e. Round block or volume displacement technique in the case of periareolar lesions

2. Reconstruction of the breast using adjacent fat tissue, for example:

    a. Quadrantectomy or hemimastectomy with a latissimus dorsi flap (case 5)

    b. Quadrantectomy or lumpectomy with thoraco-epigastric flap (rarely used), (case 6)

5.1 Case 1

5.1.1 Description of case 1

The tumor is located in the upper inner quadrant (**Figure 1a**). First, the tumor is resected with the skin over the tumor bed (**Figure 1b**). The status after resection of the full thickness arriving at the major pectoralis muscle is shown in **Figure 1c**. After that, the skin in the axillary area is removed (**Figure 1d**). This step can also be done at the beginning when the sentinel lymph node should be removed. Then, the tissue is mobilized medially, and the flap is remodeled in the defect area (**Figure 1e** and **f**). As a last step, the skin incision is extended to perform the mastopexy in order to recentralize the nipple-areolar complex (NAC) (**Figure 1g**). Finally, the wound is sutured with 3.0 Monocryl running sub- and intracutaneously (**Figure 1h**).

Figure 2a shows how the skin and flap tissue are medially mobilized after resection of the tumor and removing of the sentinel lymph node. For a better symmetry, the incision is extended to realize a mastopexy (**Figure 2b**).

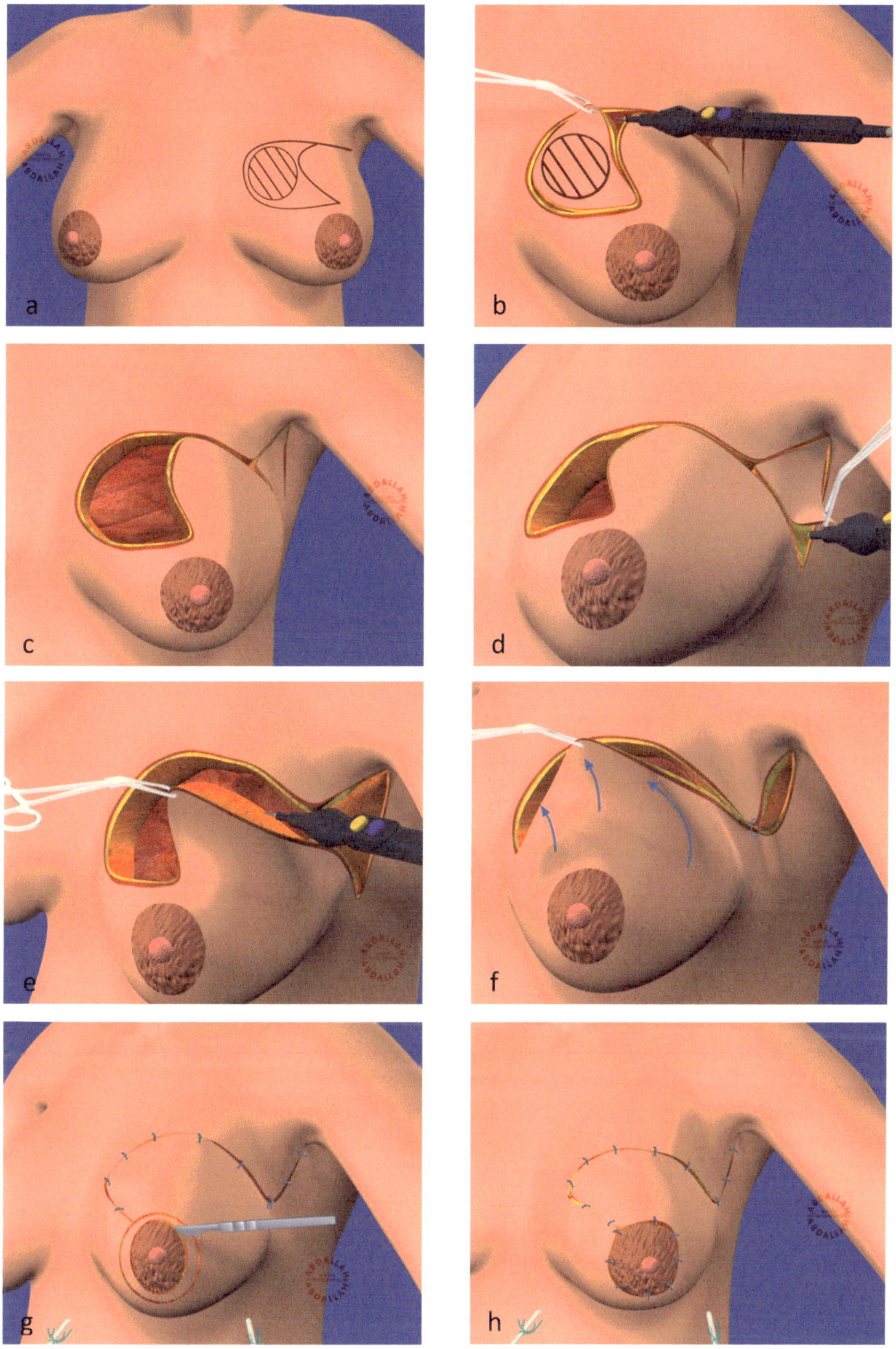

Figure 1.
Step-by-step illustration of tumor resection in the upper inner quadrant followed by reconstruction with a rotational flap.

Figure 2c presents the status after the adaptation of the wound and performance of a mastopexy for better optimization. The postoperative result is shown in **Figure 2d**.

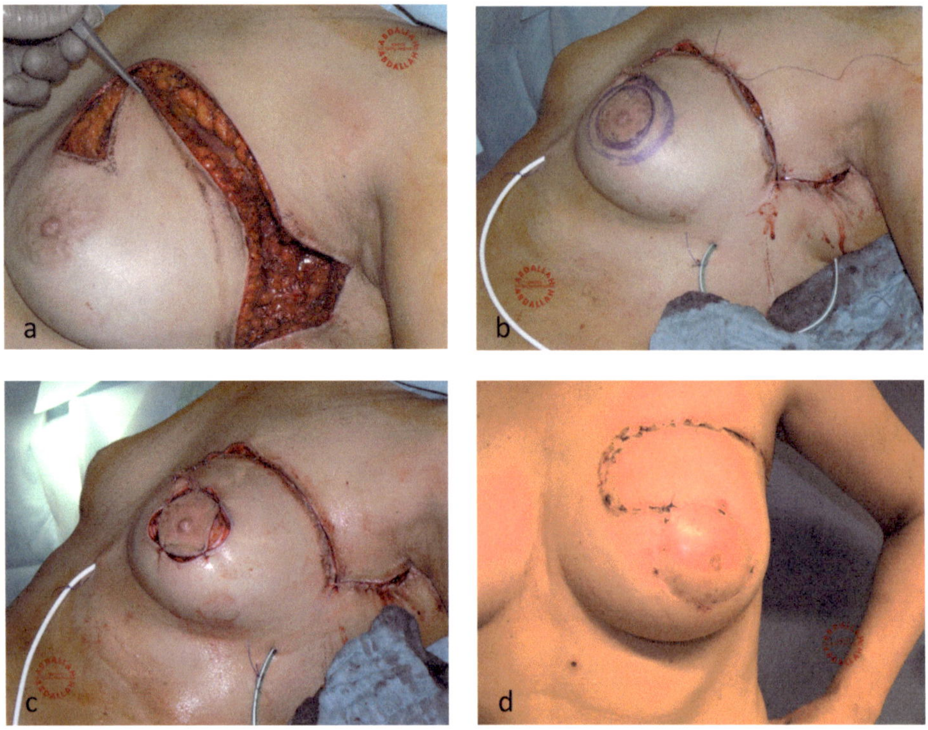

Figure 2.
Intraoperative photos and the postoperative result after resection of the tumor in the upper inner quadrant.

5.2 Case 2

5.2.1 Description of case 2

In this case, the tumor is located in the right inner quadrant around 4 o'clock (**Figures 3a** and **4a**). In order to gain additional tissue from the caudal area and to increase the volume of the flap, the incision line is performed 1.5 cm under the inframammary fold (**Figures 3b** and **4a**). After the incision along the marking, the tumor is resected together with the skin leaving a huge defect in the medial area (**Figures 3c** and **4b**). Following tumor resection, the gland tissue is mobilized from the pectoral fascia cranially until the level of the NAC (**Figure 3d**). The extent of mobilization is well shown in **Figure 3e**. Then, the skin over the inframammary fold is removed permitting to rotate the caudal part of the flap inwardly and consequently to gain more volume (**Figure 3e** and **f**). The flap is rotated in the medial area to fill the defect (**Figure 3g**). Finally, the NAC is recentralized after adaptation of the wound (**Figure 3h**). The postoperative outcome is shown in **Figure 4c** and **d** [28].

5.3 Case 3

5.3.1 Description of case 3

Figure 5a shows the preoperative drawing that is usually used in the case of a tumor-adapted reduction mammoplasty. The operation starts with the resection of the NAC and the whole tissue thickness underneath it to the muscle (**Figures 5b** and **6a**). An important issue to be considered at this time of the operation is to leave all around a minimum of 0.5 cm chorion when removing the NAC bloc so that the future areola sits

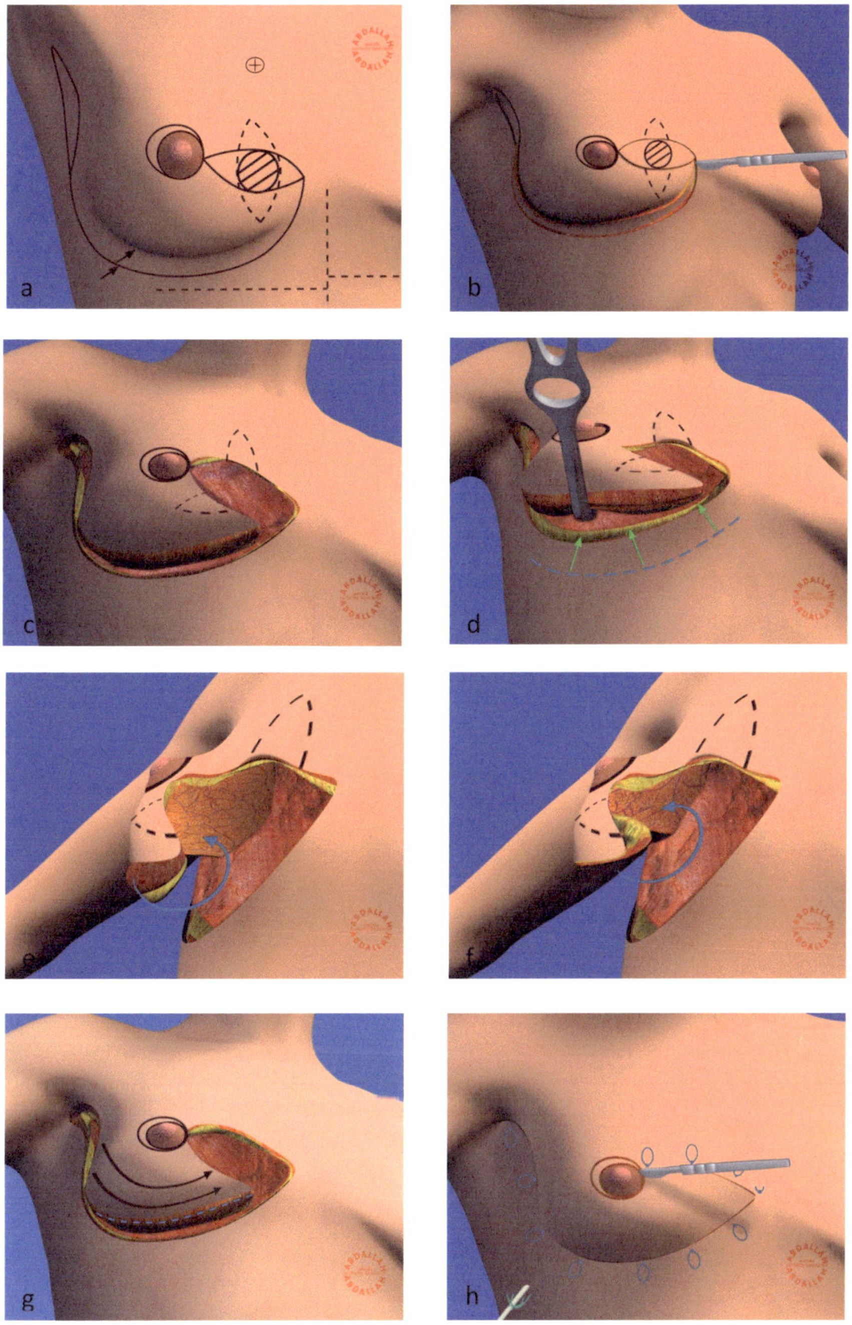

Figure 3.
Step-by-step illustration of tumor resection in the inner quadrant followed by reconstruction with a rotational flap.

on it (tip) (**Figures 5c** and **6b**). Then, the preparation of the flap will be started. The surgeon needs to perform a deepithelization of the skin leaving a skin island, which will be the newly formed areola (**Figure 6c**). After that, the flap is mobilized medially, laterally, and caudally (**Figure 5d** and **e**). At this level, the flap is only basally stalked (**Figure 5f**). Finally, both sides of the wound are adapted (**Figure 6d**), and the final result will be as shown in **Figure 6e** and **f**. The areola position is supported through the left chorion. Otherwise, the NAC can sink into the defect area.

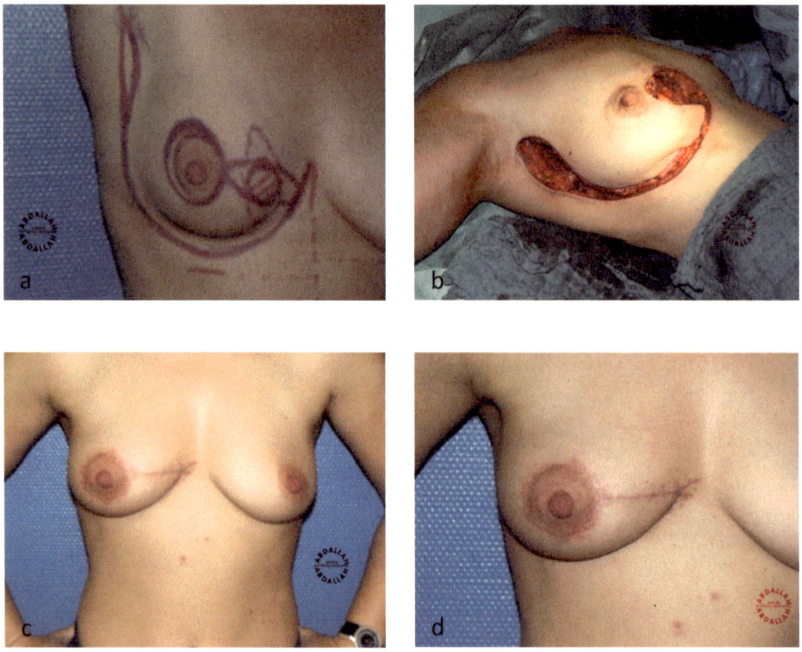

Figure 4.
Intraoperative photos and the postoperative result after resection of the tumor in the inner quadrant.

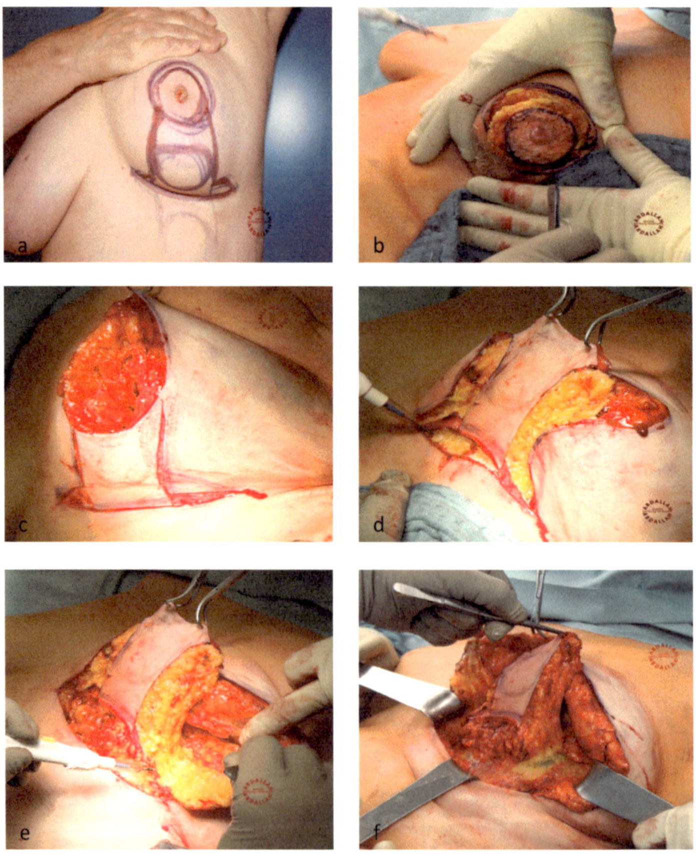

Figure 5.
Intraoperative photos illustrating the steps of tumor-adapted reduction mammoplasty (a–f).

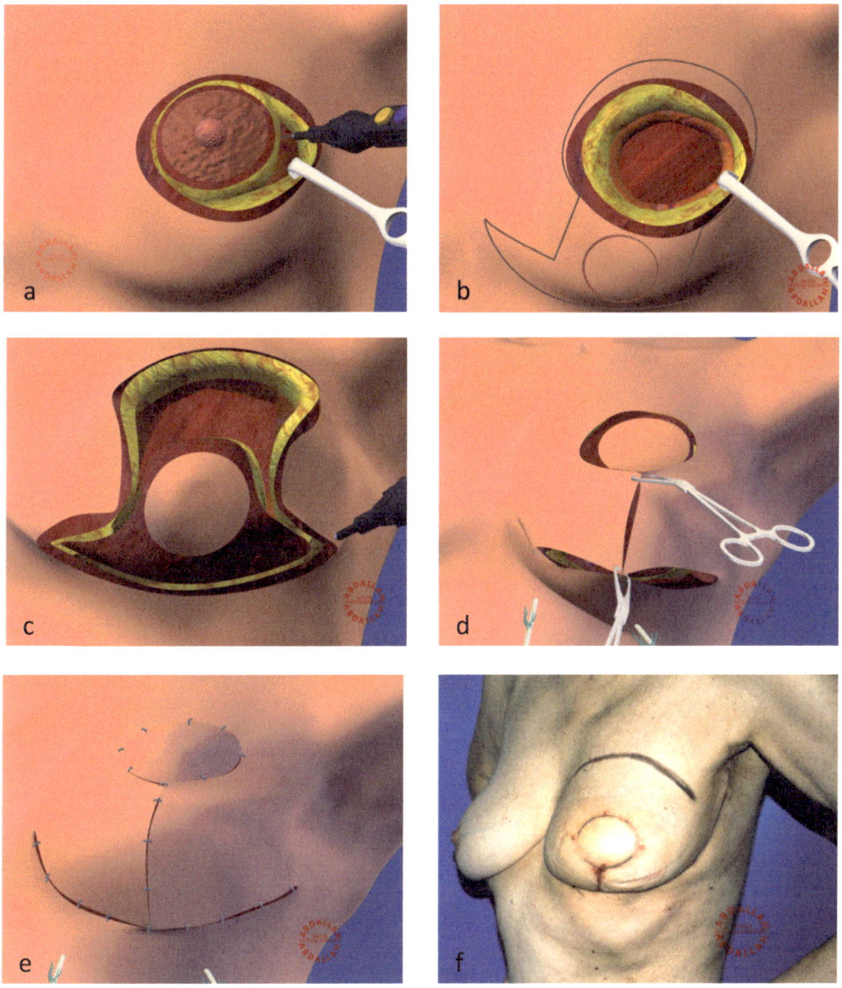

Figure 6.
Illustration of central resection and remodeling of the breast using a flap from the caudal area. Postoperative outcome is shown in (f).

5.4 Case 4

5.4.1 Description of case 4

The tumor location and the preoperative incision marking are shown in **Figure 7a** and **b** (front and side). The previously marked area is resected leaving a defect in the breast segment where the tumor was located (**Figure 7c** and **d**). After removing the tumor, the breast tissue is mobilized from the caudal as well as the axillary area to fill the defect. Both sides of the wound are adapted together. The reshaping of the breast is completed by performing a mastopexy to recentralize the nipple-areolar complex.

5.5 Case 5

5.5.1 Description of case 5

In this case, the patient first received a breast-conserving surgery for breast cancer on the right side. The initial tumor was resected in free margins. On the

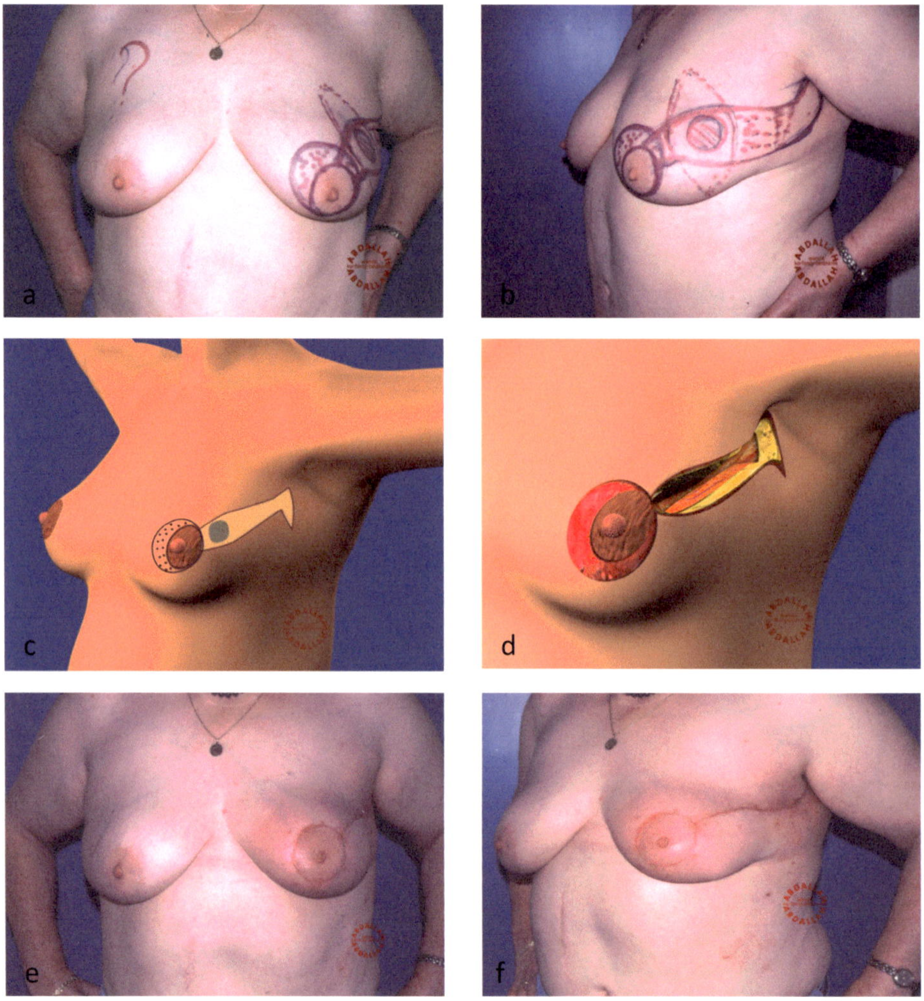

Figure 7.
Drawings of tumor resection in the left upper outer quadrant with the postoperative outcome.

final pathology, ductal carcinoma in situ (DCIS) components were incidentally found on the lateral margins making the first surgery a R1-resection. A hemimastectomy was indicated to ensure a R0-resection. The extension of the resection is shown in **Figure 8a** and **b**. The incision marking on the back is shown in **Figure 8c** and **d**. After the hemimastectomy, the fat tissue is mobilized and separated from the lateral thoracic wall arriving at the latissimus muscle edge (**Figure 8e** and **f**). Then, the latissimus skin and fat island with the underlying muscle is mobilized and transposed in the breast defect area (**Figure 8g**). After fixation of the mobilized caudal tissue on the major pectoral muscle, the flap is adapted to the wound edges (**Figure 8h**). The postoperative result was as shown in **Figure 9a** and **b** [28].

5.6 Case 6

5.6.1 Description of case 6

In this case, the patient has previously received breast-conserving surgery followed with radiotherapy for breast cancer. She presented at our clinic for a defect in the

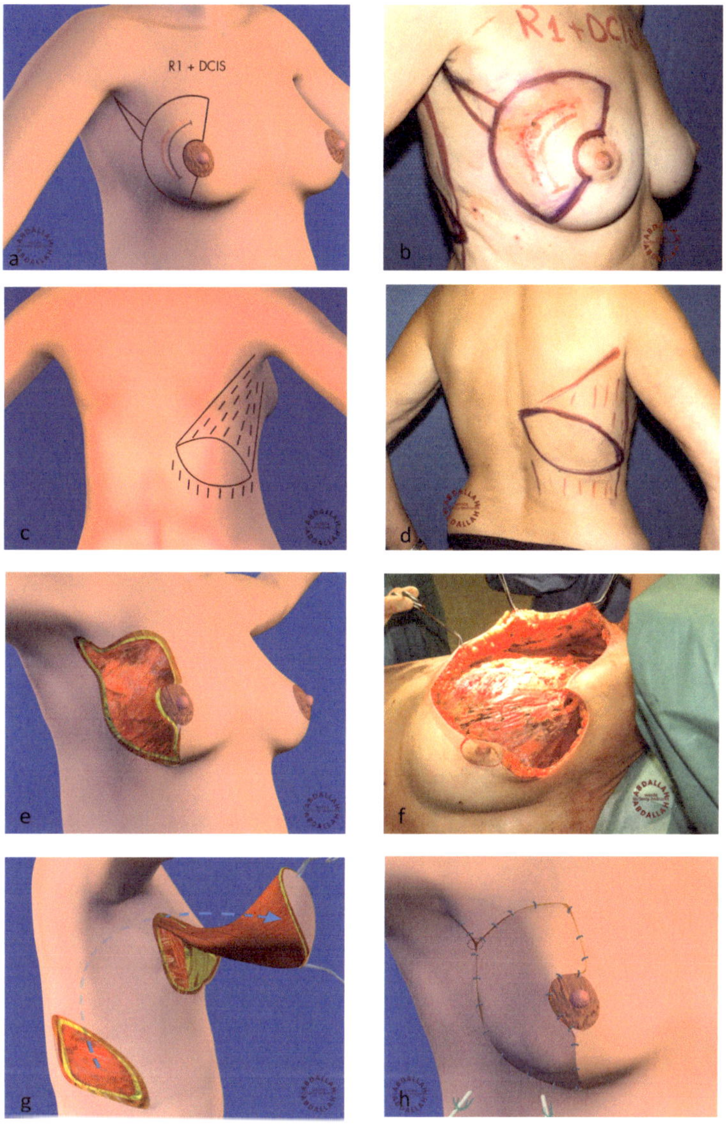

Figure 8.
Step-by-step illustration of a right hemimastectomy followed by reconstruction with a latissimus dorsi flap.

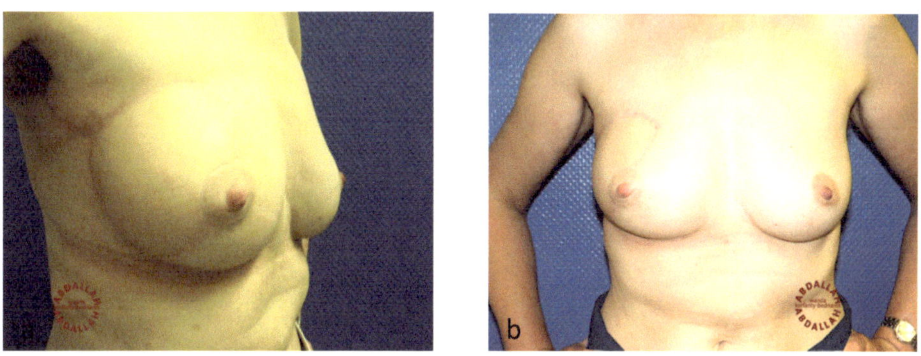

Figure 9.
Postoperative outcome after reconstruction of the hemimastectomy defect with a latissimus dorsi muscle flap.

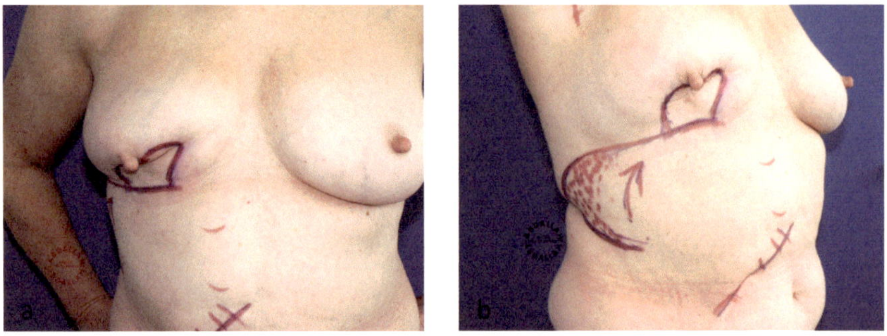

Figure 10.
Preoperative incision drawing in a patient presenting a defect in the inferior quadrant after receiving a breast-conserving surgery and radiotherapy for breast cancer.

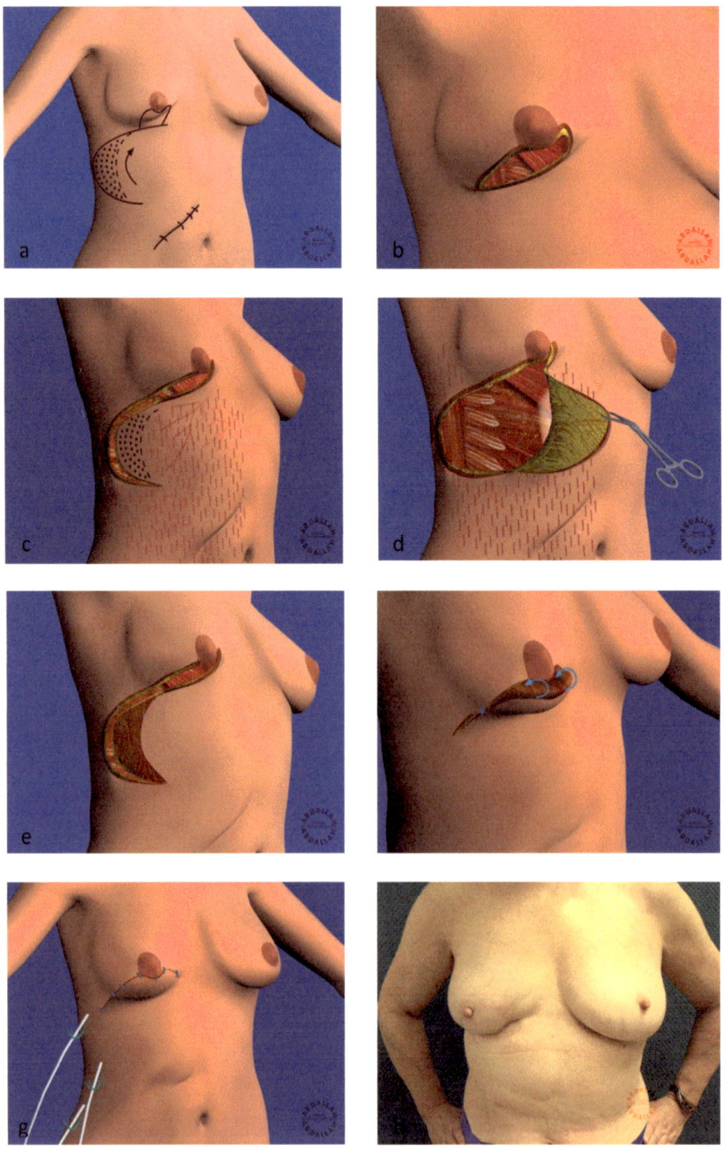

Figure 11.
Step-by-step illustration of reconstruction of lower breast defect with a thoraco-epigastric flap.

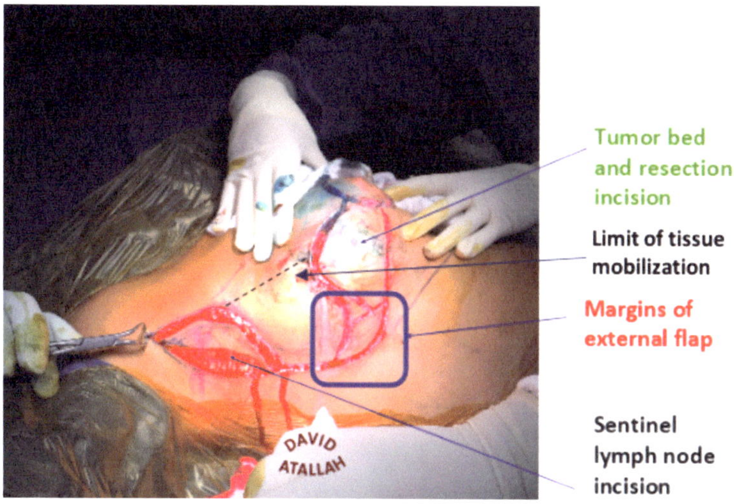

Figure 12.
Tumor located at the union of outer quadrants and using the lateral fat to fill the defect. An intraoperative photo showing the resection incision, the borders of the lateral fat flap to be used as well as the incision for the sentinel lymph node.

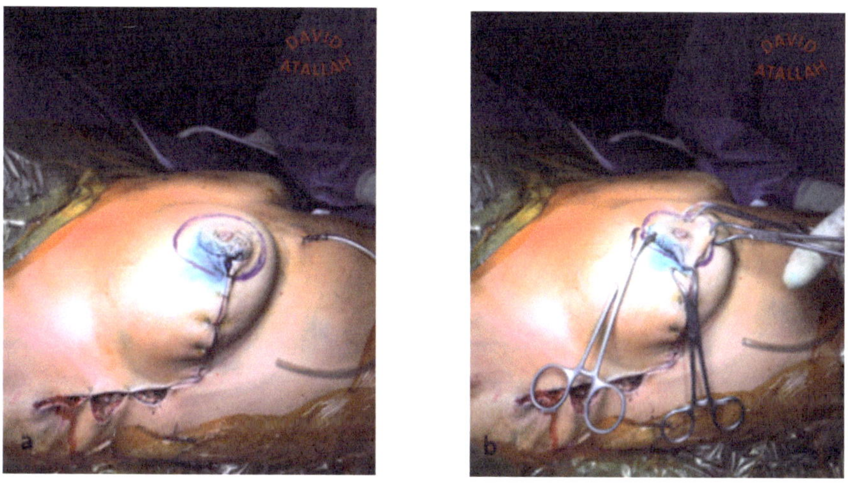

Figure 13.
An intraoperative photo showing the status after remodeling of the breast and adaptation of the wound. The drawing of the mastopexy and the checking of the mastopexy limits using Backhaus towel clamps are shown in **Figure 14a** *and* **b***, respectively.*

operation area accompanied with pain. She was planned for removal of the scarred tissue and defect coverage with a thoraco-epigastric flap. The drawings in **Figure 10a** and **b** show the breast area to be removed and also the flap that needs to be mobilized. The lower marked scar is an old open cholecystectomy scar (**Figure 11a**). First, the scarred area is removed as shown in **Figure 11b**. Second, the incision is extended laterally and then inferiorly as preoperatively marked permitting to harvest the intended flap (**Figure 11c**). Then, the upper abdominal flap is mobilized and separated from the abdominal wall. The scar of the cholecystectomy is as well dissected. The red dots show the extension of the mobilization (**Figure 11d**). The black dots show the skin area which is deepithelialized and inserted in the wound area (**Figure 11c** and **e**). The flap is transposed, and the deepithelialized area is inserted in the defective areal and fixed on

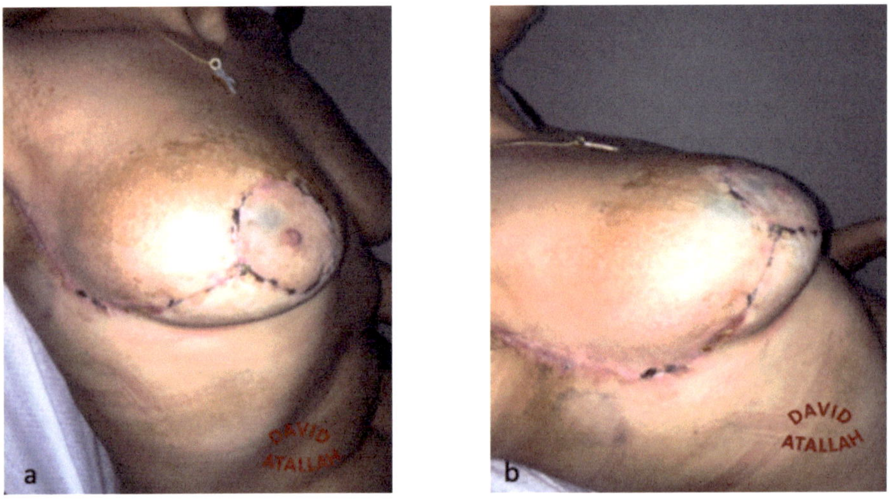

Figure 14.
Postoperative outcome after outer quadrant breast resection and reconstruction using oncoplastic technique.

the pectoral fascia (**Figure 11f**). The status after adaptation of the wound and postoperative result are shown in **Figure 11g** and **h** [28].

5.7 Case 7

5.7.1 Description of the case

In this case, we want to raise the attention on the importance of sparing every centimeter of fat tissue that could be used and mobilized when trying to fill the defect created after a wide breast excision.

After resection of the tumor, we can use an external fat flap that will be deepithelialized and then mobilized internally to contribute to a better form of the remodeled breast (**Figure 12**). The flap is mobilized internally and then covered by both glandular pillars (superior and inferior) (**Figure 13a**). In the last step, the NAC is recentralized using mastopexy (**Figure 13b**). The postoperative result after 2 weeks is as shown in **Figure 14a** and **b**.

6. Complications

Massive breast mobilization and recentralization of the nipple during oncoplastic surgery cause tissue trauma, large wound surfaces, and surgical dead space, which may increase the risk of complications [29].

First, some complications are frequently seen after an oncoplastic surgery. Actually, the manipulation and mobilization of the breast may compromise the blood supply of flap tissue and make it prone to present fat necrosis in 5% of cases. Sometimes the fat necrosis may impair the ability to adequately screen for tumor recurrence and can be mistaken for a suspicious lesion or local recurrence which may require more tissue sampling procedures in order to rule out malignancy [30]. In addition, seroma formation is commonly seen after oncoplastic surgery. The presence of seroma may also delay the delivery of adjuvant therapy and may be seen in 8–10% of cases. Wound healing can also be protracted in patients receiving oncoplastic surgery in comparison to standard surgery especially in the case of smoking history. Moreover, asymmetry can also be an issue after oncoplasty [31]. However, an adjustment of the contralateral side can always be offered especially when the size difference between the two sides is remarkable. Also, there is a risk of nipple malposition in the case of lack of mastopexy when needed. Loss of nipple sensitivity can occur and may be related not only to nipple-areolar complex manipulation but also to radiotherapy effect.

Second, other complications can occur after oncoplasty but may rarely be observed. For example, partial nipple necrosis or complete nipple loss can be a devastating complication for both the patient and surgeon in 0.5% of cases. That is why it is essential to select wisely the patients, the safest possible technique, and encourage them to reduce risk factors. In the case of very thin flaps, skin necrosis can be expected. The radiotherapy after the oncoplastic surgery can occasionally lead to breast deformity especially in the case of mostly fatty very-low-density breasts. Patients with smoking history, uncontrolled diabetes, or postoperative infection are prone to develop breast fibrosis.

Last but not the least, special concern should be made when combining oncoplastic surgery with intraoperative radiotherapy because these cases were associated with a high risk of fat necrosis in our patients collectively. Also, a particular attention should be given when operating slim women with small breasts. Due to the small available volume, the reshaping of the breast cannot be sufficient resulting in deformity and NAC malposition.

7. Conclusion

The introduction of oncoplastic surgery has helped to optimize esthetic outcomes in breast cancer management without compromising oncological safety. Along with wider volume resection, this technique can also maintain breast shape and appearance. Indeed, an excellent postoperative outcome starts with a preoperative planning done by an experienced surgeon who will take into consideration the breast volume, tumor size and location, breast density, and patient's age and comorbidities. It is not a one technique fits all, but it is about the capability of blending art and science in every case individually based on the mentioned principles.

Author details

Atallah David[1*], Moubarak Malak[1] and Abdallah Abdallah[2]

1 Hôtel-Dieu de France University Hospital, Saint Joseph University, Beirut, Lebanon

2 Evangelische Kliniken, Gelsenkirchen, Germany

*Address all correspondence to: david.atallah@gmail.com

References

[1] Halsted WS. The results of operations for the cure of cancer of the breast performed at the Johns Hopkins Hospital from June, 1889, to January, 1894. Annals of Surgery. 1894;**20**:497-555

[2] Patey DH, Dyson WH. The prognosis of carcinoma of the breast in relation to the type of operation performed. British Journal of Cancer. 1948;**2**:7-13

[3] Veronesi U, Saccozzi R, Del Vecchio M, et al. Comparing radical mastectomy with quadrantectomy, axillary dissection, and radiotherapy in patients with small cancers of the breast. The New England Journal of Medicine. 1981;**305**:6-11

[4] Fisher B, Bauer M, Margolese R, et al. Five-year results of a randomized clinical trial comparing total mastectomy and segmental mastectomy with or without radiation in the treatment of breast cancer. The New England Journal of Medicine. 1985;**312**(11):665-673

[5] Acea B. Cirugía oncológica de la mama. In: Técnicas Oncoplásticas y Reconstructivas. Spain: Elsevier; 2018

[6] Silverstein M, Mai T, Savalia N, Vaince F, Guerra L. Oncoplastic breast conservation surgery: The new paradigm. Journal of Surgical Oncology. 2014;**110**(1):82-89

[7] Clough KB, Soussaline M, Campana F, Salmon RJ. Mammoplasty combined with irradiation: Conservative treatment of cancers located in the lower quadrants. Annales de Chirurgie Plastique et Esthétique. 1990;**35**(2):117-122

[8] Cothier-Savey I, Otmezguine Y, Calitchi E, et al. Value of reduction mammoplasty in the conservative treatment of breast neoplasm. A propos of 70 cases. Annales de Chirurgie Plastique et Esthétique. 1996;**41**(4):346-353

[9] Petit JY, Rietjens M, Garusi C, et al. Integration of plastic surgery in the course of breast-conserving surgery for cancer to improve results and radicality of tumor excision. Recent Results in Cancer Research. 1998;**152**:202-211

[10] Spear SL, Pelletiere CV, Wolfe AJ, et al. Experience with reduction mammoplasty combined with breast conservation therapy in the treatment of breast cancer. Plastic and Reconstructive Surgery. 2002;**111**(3):1102-1109

[11] Clough K, Kaufman G, Claude N, Buccimazza I, Sarfati I. Improving breast cancer surgery: A classification and quadrant per quadrant atlas for oncoplastic surgery. Annals of Surgical Oncology. 2010;**17**(5):1375-1391

[12] Bulstrode NW, Shortri S. Prediction of cosmetic outcome following conservative breast surgery using breast volume measurements. Breast. 2001;**10**:124-126

[13] Sakorafa s GH. Breast cancer surgery–historical evolution, current status and future perspectives. Acta Oncologica. 2001;**40**:5-18

[14] Kau r N, Petit JY, Rietjens M, Maff ini F, Luini A, Gatti G, et al. Comparative study of surgical margins in oncoplastic surgery and quadrantectomy in breast cancer. Annals of Surgical Oncology. 2005;**12**:1-7

[15] Urban C, Lima R, Schunemann E, Spautz C, Rabinovich I. Oncoplastic principles in breast conserving surgery. Breast. 2011;**20**:S92-S95

[16] Hollingsworth AB, Stough RG, O'Dell CA, et al. Breast magnetic resonance imaging for preoperative locoregional staging. American Journal of Surgery. 2008;**196**:389-397

[17] Berg WA, Gutierrez L, NessAiver MS, et al. Diagnostic accuracy of mammography, clinical examination, US, and MR imaging in preoperative assessment of breast cancer. Radiology. 2004;**233**:830-849

[18] Pediconi F, Catalano C, Padula S, et al. Contrast-enhanced magnetic resonance mammography: Does it affect surgical decision-making in patients with breast cancer? Breast Cancer Research and Treatment. 2007;**106**:65-74

[19] Barchie M, Clive K, Tyler J, Sutcliffe J, Kirkpatrick A, Bell L, et al. Standardized pretreatment breast MRI-accuracy and influence on mastectomy decisions. Journal of Surgical Oncology. 2011;**104**(7):741-745

[20] Houssami N, Ciatto S, Macaskill P, et al. Accuracy and surgical impact of magnetic resonance imaging in breast cancer staging: Systematic review and meta-analysis in detection of multifocal and multicentric cancer. Journal of Clinical Oncology. 2008;**26**(19):3248-3258

[21] Jochelson MS, Lampen-Sachar K, Gibbons G, Dang C, Lake D, Morris EA, et al. Do MRI and mammography reliably identify candidates for breast conservation after neoadjuvant chemotherapy. Annals of Surgical Oncology. 2015;**22**(5):1490-1495

[22] Halpern EF, Niklason LT. Assessing radiologist performance using combined digital mammography and breast tomosynthesis compared with digital mammography alone: Results of a multicenter, multireader trial. Radiology. 2013;**266**:104-113

[23] Ciatto S, Houssami N, Bernardi D, Caumo F, Pellegrini M, Brunelli S, et al. Integration of 3D digital mammography with tomosynthesis for population breast-cancer screening (STORM): A prospective comparison study. The Lancet Oncology. 2013;**14**:583-589

[24] Skaane P, Bandos AI, Gullien R, Eben EB, Ekseth U, Haakenaasen U, et al. Comparison of digital mammography alone and digital mammography plus tomosynthesis in a population-based screening program. Radiology. 2013;**267**:47-56

[25] Krammer J, Stepniewski K, Kaiser C, Brade J, Riffel P, Schoenberg S, et al. Value of additional digital breast tomosynthesis for preoperative staging of breast cancer in dense breasts. Anticancer Research. 2017;**37**(9):5255-5261

[26] Mall S, Lewis S, Brennan P, Noakes J, Mello-Thoms C. The role of digital breast tomosynthesis in the breast assessment clinic: A review. Journal of Medical Radiation Sciences. 2017;**64**(3):203-211

[27] Margenthaler J. Optimizing conservative breast surgery. Journal of Surgical Oncology. 2011;**103**(4):306-312

[28] Abdallah A. Oncoplastic Breast Surgery: Case-Related Atlas. Cologne, Germany: Deutscher Ärzte-Verlag GmbH; 2009

[29] Weber W, Soysal S, Fulco I, Barandun M, Babst D, Kalbermatten D, et al. Standardization of oncoplastic breast conserving surgery. European Journal of Surgical Oncology. 2017;**43**(7):1236-1243

[30] Losken A, Schaefer TG, Newell M, Stybl OT. The impact of partial breast reconstruction using reduction techniques on post-operative cancer surveillance. Plastic and Reconstructive Surgery. 2009;**124**:9-17

[31] Bertozzi N, Pesce M, Santi P, Raposio E. Oncoplastic breast surgery: Comprehensive review. European Review for Medical and Pharmacological Sciences. 2017;**21**(11):2572-2525

Section 3

Breast Reconstruction

Chapter 7

Breast Reconstruction with TRAM Flap

Ercan Karacaoglu

Abstract

Traditional breast conservative therapy (BCT) is lumpectomy, sentinel lymph node biopsy and possible axillary dissection, and radiation therapy. BCT is, as known and considered all over the world, is oncologically equivalent to mastectomy with regard to overall long-term survival rates. BCT is the recommended treatment of choice for women with early stages breast cancer. The main philosophy of BCT is optimizing cosmetic goals and minimizing the psychological morbidity of a mastectomy while ensuring low rates of local recurrence. Achieving an oncologically safe resection is maintained by tumor margin clearance. Ensuring an oncologic clearance with increasing tumor size requires extensive breast parenchyma resection. And this results in large volume resection and this requires volume replacement techniques. Depending on the amount of breast volume resected, an autologous tissue transfer may be required to achieve requirement of breast restoration. Latissimus dorsi flap and TRAM flap are two autologous tissues mostly used to fulfill this restoration. This chapter focuses on the TRAM flap, one of the most commonly used autologous tissue in volume replacement reconstruction of the mastectomy defect.

Keywords: TRAM, flap, breast, reconstruction, pediculated, skin sparing, mastectomy, autologous, repair

1. Introduction

Breast reconstruction with transverse rectus abdominis myocutaneous (TRAM) flap has its own unique features and requirements. Not all cases require TRAM flap, and TRAM flap is not the best option for every case. That can be analyzed by comparing available treatment options of breast cancer (or breast deformities) and reconstruction.

Traditional breast conservative therapy (BCT) is lumpectomy, sentinel lymph node biopsy, possible axillary dissection, and radiation therapy. BCT, as known and considered all over the world, is oncologically equivalent to mastectomy with regard to overall long-term survival rates. BCT is the recommended treatment of choice for women with early stages of breast cancer [1, 2]. The main philosophy of BCT is optimizing cosmetic goals and minimizing the psychological morbidity of a mastectomy while ensuring low rates of local recurrence.

Achieving an oncologically safe resection is maintained by tumor margin clearance [2]. Ensuring an oncologic clearance with increasing tumor size requires extensive breast parenchyma resection. And this results in large volume resection, and this requires volume replacement techniques. Depending on the amount of breast volume resected, an autologous tissue transfer may be required to achieve requirement of breast restoration. Latissimus dorsi flap and TRAM flap are two autologous tissues mostly used to fulfill this restoration. Perforator flaps are also available within the last two decades, and some centers and surgeons began to use them as the procedure of choice. This chapter focuses on the TRAM flap, one of the most commonly used autologous tissue in volume replacement reconstruction of the mastectomy defect.

The results of breast reconstruction have improved dramatically over the past 30 years. The main reason for this improvement is the experience that has grown from various techniques of flap surgery. Breast reconstruction entered the modern era with the introduction of the TRAM flap in 1982 by Hartrampf et al. [3]. This ingenious procedure reliably transfers autogenous tissue from the lower abdomen for breast reconstruction. This surgery has also the added benefit of abdominal rejuvenation.

2. Pertinent anatomy

The adult female breast lies with its footprint extending from the second to sixth ribs. The medial border is at the edge of the sternum, and the lateral border is at the anterior axillary line. The female breast has a circular shape except the upper outer quadrant, where the axillary tail of Spence extends to the armpit. The breast is a modified cutaneous gland. The mature breast demonstrates both a superficial and a deep fascia support system. From an embryological standpoint, the breast bud develops within the Scarpa's fascia. This fascia splits to form anterior and posterior lamella. Anterior lamella serves as a dissection plane for surgeons when performing a mastectomy, while the posterior lamella separates the breasts from the underlying pectoralis major muscle. Breast duct network often extends more widely than this footprint. In about 15% of cases, breast tissue extends below the costal margin. It is critical when performing breast reconstruction that the inframammary fold (IMF) is maintained or at least identified and reconstructed if surgical removal of additional breast tissue below this fold is required [4–6]. The breast lobule is the basic unit of the breast. Each breast consists of roughly 20 lobules. The breast has its breast duct network starting from acini or alveoli, excretory duct, and lactiferous duct. A total of 15–20 lactiferous ducts drain the entire breast and dilate into the milk sinus beneath the areola. The stroma within the breast consists of connective tissue, nerves, blood vessels, and lymphatic channels.

Arterial supply: The blood supply of the breast is diffuse and comes from a variety of potential sources including internal mammary artery, lateral thoracic artery, branches from thoracoacromial artery, and intercostal arteries. *The internal mammary artery system* has both deep and superficial blood supplies and provides more than half of total breast blood flow by anterior and posterior perforating branches. *The lateral thoracic vessels* have both dermal and dermoglandular pedicles with adequate both arterial input and venous drainage [5]. *Minor sources of arterial supply* to the breast are posterior intercostal arteries (third, fourth, and fifth) and branches from the axillary artery, the thoracic artery, the subscapular artery, and the pectoralis branches of the thoracoacromial artery.

Venous drainage: The venous drainage of the breast is superficial and deep. The superficial system has transverse and longitudinal veins. The deep system empties into internal mammary vein, axillary vein, and perforating branches of posterior intercostal veins [5].

Arterial inflow is strong enough to support blood supply, but venous return is also a key in designing and avoiding congestion and increasing the security of the perfusion of both breast parenchyma and skin envelopes. This is one of the key issues for the viable results in breast oncologic surgery and in breast reconstruction.

Lymphatic drainage: The lymphatic drainage of the breast is also diffuse and variable. Traditionally recognized lymphatic basins include the axillary nodes as well as nodes along the internal mammary vessels.

Innervation: The innervation of the breast is also diffuse and variable. Multiple nerve branches from the lateral and anterior cutaneous branches of the second through the sixth intercostal nerves as well as the supraclavicular nerves enter and branch within the breast. The lateral branches are more significant than the smaller anterior branches.

2.1 Basic anatomy for tram flap

Rectus abdominis muscle: The rectus abdominis muscles are pairs of long, straight muscles that flex the spine and tighten the intra-abdominal wall. This muscle has its origin from the symphysis pubis and the pubic crest and inserts on the linea alba and the fifth, sixth, and seventh costal cartilages. Each muscle has two to five tendinous inscriptions. The most caudal inscription is at the level of umbilicus. These tendinous inscriptions are not adherent to the posterior sheath but to overlying anterior rectus sheath. Rectus sheath is thick and encloses the rectus abdominis muscle except for the posterior part below the arcuate line. The arcuate line is mostly located halfway between the umbilicus and symphysis pubis. The arcuate line is the transition point where the internal oblique aponeurosis stops to split and the aponeurosis of all three muscles pass ventral to the rectus abdominis muscle. Below the arcuate line, there is only the transversalis fascia where this is the region of weakness and it is the place potential herniation after flap dissection. The linea alba is the decussation of the fused aponeurosis in the midline. The linea alba is wider close to the xiphoid process and narrows to a fine a line below the umbilicus. The lateral border of the rectus muscle with its sheath is referred to as the linea semilunaris.

Blood supply: The blood supply to the rectus muscle and TRAM flap comes from the deep superior epigastric artery (DSEA), which arises from the internal thoracic (mammary) artery, and the deep inferior epigastric artery (DIEA), a branch of the external iliac artery. Both the deep superior and inferior epigastric arteries communicate within the rectus abdominis muscle and the overlying muscular and cutaneous tissue of the anterior abdominal wall. The DSEA and DIEA systems connect above the umbilicus through a system of small-caliber vessels that Taylor and Palmer refer to as "choke" vessels [7]. The DIEA originates approximately 1 cm above the inguinal ligament and then pierces the transversalis fascia and enters the rectus sheath just below the arcuate line. The DIEA then ascends obliquely and medially between the rectus abdominis muscle and the posterior wall of the rectus sheath. The DIEA divides into two or three large branches below the level of the umbilicus. It shows certain type of arborization, extensive studies reported by Moon and Taylor. Based on their outcomes, there are three types of anastomosis between DIEA and DSEA. Most patients have two networks (57%), while there are three networks in 14% of the people and only one major anastomosis in 29% of the people [8].

Perforators are key for the vascular supply of TRAM flap. These vessels are terminal branches of the DIEA and deep inferior epigastric veins. Perforators extend from the vertical epigastric system and pass through the anterior rectus sheath, supplying the skin and subcutaneous tissue. Taylor and Palmer studies demonstrated a rich connection between the DIEA system and the abdominal wall skin. The majority of perforators are between the umbilicus and the arcuate line, but the highest concentration of perforators is in the periumbilical area. Usually there are two parallel rows of perforators, a medial one and a lateral one. Incorporation of the periumbilical perforators permits the harvesting of a skin flap with virtually any orientation from the midline [9, 10].

TRAM flap can be planned either unipedicled or bipedicled. The decision about pedicle depends on the requirement of the tissue pad to be transferred. If a surgeon needs almost up to 60% of the lower abdominal tissue, then unipedicle might be the right choice. If the requirement is more than that, then it would be better to go with bipedicled flap.

3. TRAM flap

Breast reconstruction with TRAM flap can be accomplished with a variety of lower abdomen flap and techniques such as pedicled TRAM flap (uni- or bipedicled), free TRAM flap, or DIEP flap. The scope of this chapter is pedicled TRAM flap.

Patient selection: The very first part of this procedure should be patient selection. The candidate should be evaluated as to the status of her disease and overall health. She should be emotionally stable. She should have a good motivation. All details regarding surgery, hospitalization, and recuperation need to be discussed in detail.

Who are candidates for TRAM flap breast reconstruction? In general speaking, mastectomy defect needs to be evaluated before planning (**Figure 1**). The best candidates are as follows:

1. Patients with large and ptotic breasts where the contralateral breast needs to be altered for symmetry purpose.

2. Patients with big mastectomy defect and/or poor skin quality due to excessive dissection, skin slough, radiation effect, etc.

The best candidates for TRAM flap harvesting are the patients with well-padded lower abdominal soft tissue and loose upper abdominal soft tissue. Patient with excessive abdominal fat might not be a good candidate [11].

Who are not candidates for TRAM flap breast reconstruction? The scar on the abdomen is also a key to analyze patient eligibility for TRAM flap. A subcostal or transverse incision that divides the rectus abdominis muscle and its superior epigastric blood supply might be a contraindication for the use of a pedicled TRAM flap. Lower abdominal incision such as Pfannenstiel incision is not a contraindication for a TRAM flap, and contrary to fact, such an incision might play a "delay phenomena" effect. Patients ideally should be nonsmoker, or if they are smoker,

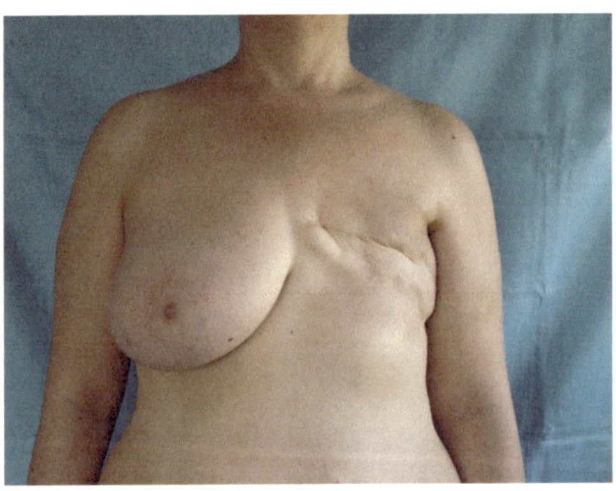

Figure 1.
Typical mastectomy defect and best candidates for breast reconstruction with TRAM flap are as seen in the picture.

they need to stop smoking almost 1–2 months before surgery. If the patient is on chemotherapy, it would be better to wait at least 6 months more after the last cure of chemotherapy. If there is a history of radiation therapy, it would be better to postpone surgery for another 6 months to year after the last cure of radiation therapy. The last condition can be totally excluded based on the recipient area requirement such as radiation-induced soft tissue defect in the mastectomy area or other soft tissue defects due to the mastectomy.

3.1 Preoperative marking and patient positioning

All markings are made with the patient in an upright standing position.

Recipient area: The inframammary, parasternal, anterior axillary line of the contralateral breast is marked. The template of these lines is reflected to the recipient side on a mirror image. The footprint of the recipient side is also copied from the contralateral breast. The marking are also made for the future inframammary fold and the tunnel that the flap would pass through (**Figure 2**).

Donor area: The TRAM flap is marked as a horizontal ellipse on the lower abdomen. Perforators around the umbilicus and below it are marked with the aid of a handheld Doppler US. The whole ellipse is tried to fit with these perforators as much as possible. The inferior incision is placed in the low bikini area. The best inferior incision location would be suprapubic crease, but this might not be possible in each case. The excursion of the lower bikini area should be tested by pinching. The superior incision line is marked 1 cm above or below the umbilicus. A superior incision that is above the umbilicus is preferable as this has a higher chance to include as much periumbilical perforators as possible. But the ease of donor area closure is the key factor to place the superior incision line (**Figure 2**).

A TRAM flap is divided into four zones based on the reliability of perfusion. There are four zones for a unipedicled TRAM flap scenario. Zone 1 refers to the skin overlying each lateral rectus abdominis muscle. Zone 2 refers to the skin overlying contralateral rectus abdominis muscle. The skin territory on each side of the

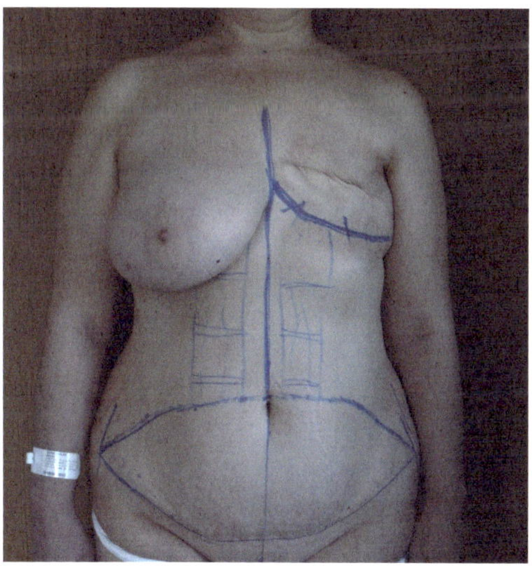

Figure 2.
Marking for the TRAM flap. All markings are made with the patient in an upright standing position. Recipient area: the inframammary, parasternal, anterior axillary line of the contralateral breast is marked. The template of these lines is reflected to the recipient side on a mirror image. Footprint of the recipient side is also copied from the contralateral breast. The marking are also made for the future inframammary crease and the tunnel that the flap would pass through.

abdomen lateral to the linea semilunaris is referred to as zone 3, and the skin lateral to the opposite linea semilunaris is zone 4. The perfusion of zones 4 and 3 is less than zones 1 and 2 where zone 4 is the most tenuous.

Surgical technique: The mastectomy skin flap is elevated off the pectoralis major muscle inferiorly and superiorly based on the preoperative marking. Previous mastectomy scar is excised and sent for pathologic evaluation.

The superior TRAM flap incision is placed till anterior rectus fascia. The upper abdominal skin flap is elevated close to both inframammary folds (IMF). A tunnel is made to the mastectomy area.

The inferior incision is placed deep to the rectus muscle, and both superficial epigastric vessels are identified and preserved. Zones 3 and 4 are dissected off the external oblique fascia, and dissection continues medially with precaution while approaching the lateral border of the rectus abdominis fascia. At this point, preoperative markings for perforators are followed, and this dissection continues medially, stopping approximately 4–5 mm lateral to these perforators. The largest perforator is mostly found just lateral and inferior to the umbilicus. An incision is made on the rectus fascia just 1 cm lateral to the perforators. The inferior epigastrics are identified easily along the lateral edge of the rectus muscle. The vessels are identified close to the external iliac artery, and the DIEA is ligated. The rectus fascia is divided vertically, and the rectus muscle with TRAM flap attached elevated off the posterior rectus fascia. The umbilicus is circumferentially incised and isolated on its stalk medially. The eight intercostal nerves are identified and transected to help for the atrophy of the muscle pedicle while approaching close to the arcus costarum. TRAM flap is delivered through the tunnel to the mastectomy site.

Anterior rectus fascia is closed with 0 or 1\0 Prolene (or nylon suture). Inferior cuff of rectus muscle is integrated to the weak area below arcuate line (**Figure 3**). Closure is reinforced with an overlay Prolene mesh that lies from epigastric area to symphysis pubis. Care must be taken not to constrict the pedicle. Abdominal skin flap is closed in layers, and the umbilicus is delivered to its new location in the midline.

The TRAM flap is provisionally placed into the mastectomy defect, and the mastectomy flap is draped over the TRAM flap. The patient is placed in a sitting position, and the TRAM flap is shaped into a breast mound. Care should be taken to shift breast mound superior and medial area to ensure adequate cleavage volume. Surely, volume distribution is important for each quadrant of breast mound (**Figures 4** and **5**).

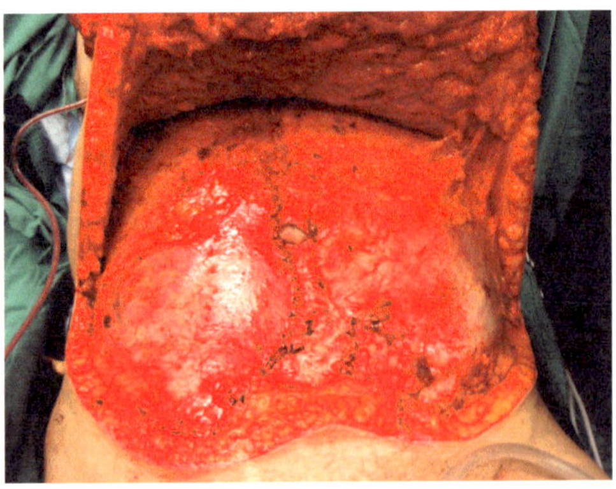

Figure 3.
Anterior rectus fascia is closed after the TRAM flap is transferred to the mastectomy site.

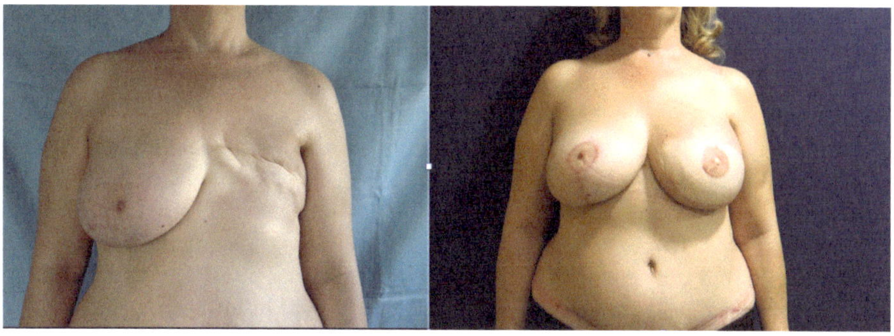

Figure 4.
Pre- and postoperative view of a mastectomy patient that is reconstructed with bipedicled TRAM flap. The patient is 56 years old. Follow-up picture was taken 6 month after nipple and areola complex reconstruction.

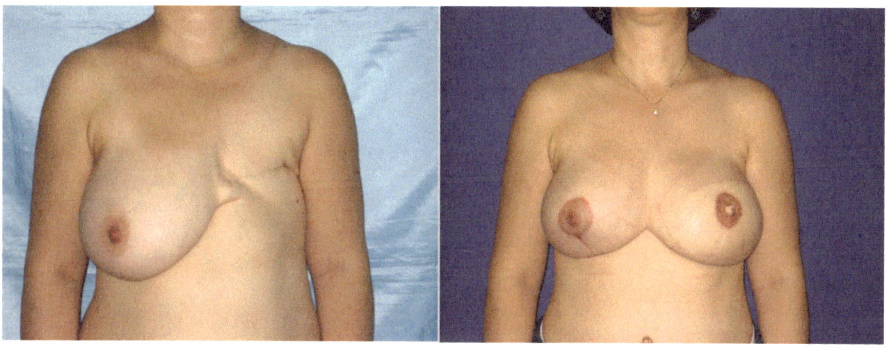

Figure 5.
Pre- and postoperative view of a mastectomy patient that is reconstructed with bipedicled TRAM flap. The patient is 48 years old.

Postoperative care: Wound care is essential, and routine wound care is needed. The flap is kept warm, and a fenestrated dressing might be a better option to observe flap perfusion. A support bra is used to maintain the position of the flap. The patient is placed in a flexed position by keeping head elevated 30° and legs elevated 20°. An abdominal girdle needs to be on at all time for 2 months. Patients are mostly hospitalized for 3 days. Patients are advised for resting for 15 days to a month after surgery.

3.2 Complications

Fat necrosis: Fat necrosis can be seen, and the reason is inadequate perfusion or limited perfusion to a certain part of the flap. Planning and surgical technique needs to be verified before and during surgery to minimize the possibility of inadequate perfusion. Planning and technique should be optimal perforator areas with limited perfusion, or question might be discarded during surgery. Zone 4 is always an area of question and must be discarded before transposing the flap.

Partial flap loss: Partial flap loss is also can be seen due to inadequate perfusion. Likewise, areas with question need to be discarded; planning and technique should be optimal to include as much perforators as possible.

Abdominal hernia: Hernia or bulging can be seen as one of the major complication. Fascial closure needs to be dome tension-free, and mesh needs to be used if indicated. Patients should be placed in abdominal girdle and told to avoid strenuous exercise till the sixth month after surgery [12]. The incidence of abdominal bulges was reported 3.8%, while hernia was reported 2.6% [13]. It is also reported that abdominal strength, as measured by the ability do sit-ups, is influenced significantly by TRAM flap.

Revisional surgeries for TRAM flap: All complications need to be revised as needed. Partial flap loss should be addressed within the first 2 weeks after surgery. Meticulous wound care is essential meanwhile.

Breast reconstruction with TRAM flap is a two-stage procedure. The goal of the first step is to reconstruct the breast mound as close as to the contralateral breast mound. The goal of the second stage is to get symmetry as much as possible and reconstruction of nipple areola complex (NAC). Surgical intervention might be needed for the contralateral breast (i.e., lifting and reduction) during the second stage. The following procedures might be done during the second stage: removal of fat necrosis, breast mound revision, IMF revision, medial cleavage revision (with flap transposition or fat grafting), donor site liposuction for feathering touch, and NAC reconstruction.

NAC reconstruction: NAC reconstruction can be done with various techniques. Some of the mostly used techniques are CV flap, skate flap, star flap, etc. Areola mostly reconstructed with pigmented full-thickness grafting from inguinal area or tattooing.

Author details

Ercan Karacaoglu
Department of Plastic Surgery, School of Medicine, Bahcesehir University, Istanbul, Turkey

*Address all correspondence to: drercanka@yahoo.com

References

[1] Veronesi U, Salvadori B, Luini A. Breast conserving is a safe method in patients with small cancer of the breast. Long-term results of three randomized trials on 1,973 patients. European Journal of Cancer. 1995;**31A**(10): 1574-1579. PMID: 7488404

[2] Fisher B, Anderson S, Redmond CK, et al. Reanalysis and results after 12 years of follow up in a randomized clinical trial comparing total mastectomy with lumpectomy with or without irradiation in the treatment of breast cancer. The New England Journal of Medicine. 1995;**333**:1456-1461. PMID: 7477145

[3] Hartrampf CR, Scheflan M, Black PW. Breast reconstruction with a transverse abdominal Island flap. Plastic and Reconstructive Surgery. 1982;**69**:216-224

[4] Evans GRD, Hall-Findlay E. History and anatomy. In: Evans GRD, Hall-Findlay E, editors. Aesthetic and Reconstructive Surgery of the Breast. China: Elsevier Saunders; 2010. pp. 1-3

[5] Hamdi M, Wuringer E, Schlenz I, Kuzbari R. Anatomy of the breast: A clinical application. In: Hamdi M, Hammond DC, Nahai F, editors. Vertical Scar Mammaplasty. Springer-Berlin Heidelberg; 2005. pp. 2-6

[6] Hammond DC, editor. Applied anatomy. In: Atlas of Aesthetic Breast Surgery. China: Elsevier Saunders; 2009. pp. 1-9

[7] Taylor G, Palmer J. The vascular territories (angiosomes) of the body: Experimental and clinical applications. British Journal of Plastic Surgery. 1987;**40**:113

[8] Bohmet H, Gabka CJ, editors. Anatomy of the transverse rectus abdominis musculocutaneous flap—The TRAM flap. In: Plastic and Reconstructive Surgery of the Breast. A Surgical Atlas. New York: George Thieme; 1997. pp. 251-258

[9] Duchateau J, Declety A, Lejour M. Innervation of the rectus abdominus muscle: Implications for rectus flaps. Plastic and Reconstructive Surgery. 1984;**82**:223

[10] Boyd JB, Taylor GI, Corlett R. The vascular territories of the superior and deep inferior epigastric systems. Plastic and Reconstructive Surgery. 1984;**73**:1

[11] Kroll SS. Why autologous tissue? Clinics in Plastic Surgery. 1998;**25**:135-143

[12] Padubidri AN, Tetman R, Browne E, Lucas A, Papay F, Larive B, et al. Complications of postmastectomy breast reconstruction in smokers, ex smokers, and nonsmokers. Plastic and Reconstructive Surgery. 2001;**107**:350-351

[13] Kroll SS, Schusterman MA, Reece GP, Miller MJ, Robb G, Evans G. Abdominal wall strength, bulging, and hernia after TRAM flap breast reconstruction. Plastic and Reconstructive Surgery. 1995;**96**(3):616-619

Chapter 8

Immediate Breast Reconstruction with Free Autologous Tissue Transfer

Justin Zelones, Suzanne Inchauste and Dung Nguyen

Abstract

Immediate breast reconstruction in the United States is increasing with the majority of patients undergoing implant-based reconstruction. The use of pedicled autologous tissues has also been used, but due to significant donor site morbidity, free autologous tissue transfer has largely replaced it. The gold standard currently for breast reconstruction is free autologous tissue transfer from the abdomen if no contraindications exist. However, not all hospitals have the expertise available to perform free autologous tissue transfers for breast reconstruction. Other donor sites available for free autologous tissue transfer include the thigh and gluteal areas. With advances in free tissue transfer techniques, the donor site morbidity and flap failure rates are minimal. The ultimate goal for any breast reconstruction patient is to achieve the appropriate size, shape, symmetry, softness, and sensation. The goal of this chapter is to assist in achieving these goals in the immediate breast reconstruction patient through the use of free autologous tissue transfers.

Keywords: breast reconstruction, autologous tissue, free flaps, deep inferior epigastric perforator, transverse rectus abdominis myocutaneous, transverse upper gracilis, profunda artery perforator, superior gluteal artery perforator,inferior gluteal artery perforator, breast ptosis, mastopexy, nipple devascularization, re-innervation, autologous with implant

1. Introduction

The incidence of mastectomy for breast cancer over the last couple decades has been increasing leading to more patients desiring breast reconstruction. While most of these patients undergo implant-based reconstruction there is a significant number of patients that have autologous reconstructions performed [1, 2]. Implant-based reconstruction is technically easier and can have good esthetic appearance but should not be used in all patients. Ideal candidates for implant-based reconstruction are those who are not obese, a non-smoker, require no radiation, and have healthy vascularized mastectomy skin flaps. Not all breast reconstruction patients meet these characteristics nor do all patients want to be subjected to secondary affects of having a foreign body used for reconstruction. More recently patients are also concerned about breast implant associated anaplastic large cell lymphoma (BIA-ALCL) [3].

The use of pedicled autologous tissue to reconstruct the breast started with the transverse rectus abdominis myocutaneous (TRAM) flap by Hartrampf in 1982 [4]. With improved understanding about perforator vascular anatomy and surgical technique, the perforator flap concept was developed. About a decade after the TRAM, the deep inferior epigastric perforator (DIEP) flap by Allen was developed, which addressed donor site morbidity by preserving muscle and fascia [5]. Another abdominal flap that uses the same skin incision and utilizes the identical skin and fat for reconstruction as the TRAM/DIEP is the superficial inferior epigastric artery (SIEA) flap but this flap requires no fascial incision. Abdominally based free flaps are the gold standard for breast reconstruction but not all patients are candidates. Patients that do not desire a scar from hip to hip or have had previous abdominoplasty, abdominal liposuction, or other significant abdominal procedures should not undergo free flaps from the abdomen for breast reconstruction. Other potential sources for autologous tissue include the thigh and gluteal areas.

The purpose of this chapter is to review the common free flaps for breast reconstruction starting from pre-operative workup to flap in-setting along with ptosis management and adjunctive intraoperative procedures.

2. Preoperative workup and flap selection

Patients that desire breast reconstruction must undergo a multidisciplinary approach utilizing a breast oncologist and plastic surgeon from a surgical standpoint and possible radiation oncologist and genetic counselor as indicated. The majority of patients undergo breast reconstruction secondary to breast cancer ablation. However, more recently there is an increase in breast reconstruction for patients desiring prophylactic mastectomies secondary to specific genetic mutations (i.e. BRCA) and/or increased risk of developing breast cancer in the future [2].

After a patient decides that she would like a mastectomy for breast cancer treatment or risk reduction, the patient will be referred to a plastic surgeon who should perform a thorough history and physical examination. The surgeon should not only discuss the risks and benefits of surgery but other alternatives to free tissue transfer breast reconstruction, which should include no reconstruction, tissue expander or implant-based reconstruction, and pedicled flap reconstruction. Possible revisional surgery should also be discussed.

The ideal breast reconstruction would involve free tissue transfer from the abdomen. Most patients in the United States have sufficient lower abdominal tissue to reconstruct a similar size breast. For thin patients with a small abdominal pannus, other sites such as the thigh or gluteal area can be used, but these are typically smaller than the abdominal tissue. In these cases other adjunctive procedures such as fat grafting, free flap stacking, and implant placement can be performed.

Most patients that undergo free tissue transfer for breast reconstruction utilize a DIEP or TRAM flap. There are various algorithms that have been proposed based on perforator size/number and flap size [6, 7]. In general, a DIEP flap can be performed for smaller flaps (<1000 g) that have adequate perforator size (>1.5 mm). Conversely, a TRAM flap is considered for larger flaps with smaller, less dominant perforators. Another abdominal flap that is used in the minority of patients is the SIEA flap. The ideal candidate for an SIEA flap is reconstruction of a small breast with a sizeable/palpable SIEA [8].

Patients that have contraindications to using the abdomen as a free tissue transfer source or who do not want the morbidity associated with these flaps can use the thigh or gluteal areas as donor sites. These flaps include the transverse upper gracilis (TUG), profunda artery perforator (PAP), and superior/inferior gluteal artery perforator (SGAP/IGAP) flaps. The benefit of these flaps is that they can be harvested unilaterally so the contralateral side can be used for later use in the future. The downfall to these flaps is that they are typically smaller than the abdominally based flaps and positioning in the operating room can be more difficult.

Some absolute contraindications to free tissue transfer breast reconstruction include the inability to undergo a lengthy procedure under general anesthesia secondary to cardiovascular/pulmonary compromise, patient desire for a less complex procedure or unwillingness to have a long donor site scar, vascular compromise of the intended flap secondary to scarring or previous surgery, and coagulopathy that cannot be controlled with medical management. Other more common relative contraindications include severe obesity [9], smoking, diabetes, end stage renal disease [10], and hemophilia/venous thromboembolism [11]. These comorbidities should be optimized prior to breast reconstruction surgery to minimize morbidity/mortality.

3. Preoperative imaging

The standard for immediate breast reconstruction is perforator flaps from the abdomen. To aid in preoperative planning and surgical technique the use of preoperative imaging has been developed. The various forms of imaging modalities to identify perforators include duplex ultrasound, computed tomographic (CT) angiography, and magnetic resonance (MR) angiography. The use of duplex ultrasound can identify the location, size, flow, and velocity of perforators from the deep inferior epigastric artery. Other benefits of duplex ultrasound are ease of use, reduced cost, and no radiation exposure when compared to CT angiography [12].

A superior imaging technique to identify perforators is the use of CT angiography, which can identify perforator size, location, and intramuscular course (**Figure 1a**). The use of CT angiography has shown to reduce operative times, improve the perfusion of flaps, and minimize donor site morbidity. Patients with previous abdominal surgeries resulting in a paramedian scar would benefit from CT angiography to assess patency of the deep inferior epigastric artery and associated perforators [12]. The ideal perforators would be large, centrally located in the flap, and have a short traverse muscular and subfascial course [13]. The sensitivity and positive predictive value of CT angiography is near 100% for locating and mapping out the course of deep inferior epigastric perforators. For patient who do not want to undergo radiation they can elect to undergo MR angiography, which can help map out the perforators but the spatial resolution is inferior to CT angiography [14].

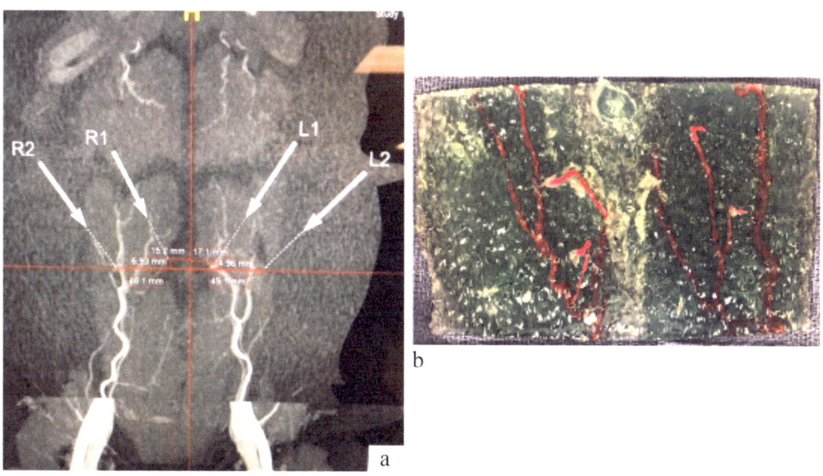

Figure 1.
(a) CT angiogram of deep inferior epigastric artery and perforators and (b) 3D model of deep inferior epigastric artery and perforators.

Our institution has developed 3D printed models of the deep inferior epigastric artery and perforators from CT angiography imaging to further aid intraoperative decision making (**Figure 1b**). The 3D printed models can be sterilized and aid in locating the larger (>1 mm) perforators in relation to the umbilicus and their course through the rectus abdominis muscle to the deep inferior epigastric artery. A limitation of the 3D printed models is their poor sensitivity to identify smaller perforators.

4. Mastectomy incisions

Surgical exposure for immediate breast reconstruction is not only dependent on flap characteristics and setup but also the choice of mastectomy incisions used. As breast cancer treatment has changed over the decades from modified radical mastectomy to nipple/skin sparing mastectomy, so have the incision choices. Traditionally, a wide elliptical incision around the NAC was performed in a transverse or oblique fashion for modified radical mastectomies. To preserve native breast skin, a circumareolar incision with or without a lateral or vertical extension can be performed resulting in a lollipop incision. A vertical extension (**Figure 2**) of a circumareolar incision is preferred over a lateral extension (**Figure 3**) as the incision can be incorporated into a mastopexy incision. Other types of mastectomy

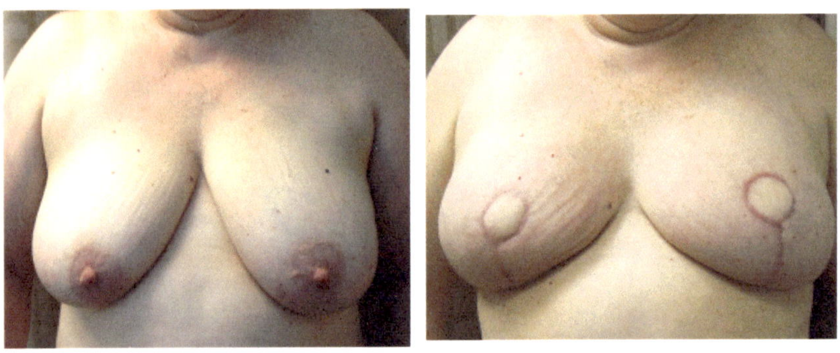

Figure 2.
TRAM flap utilizing circumareolar incision with vertical extension before and after surgery.

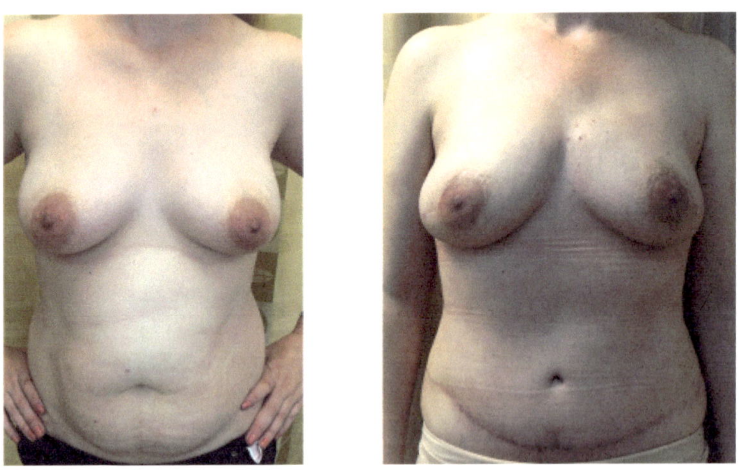

Figure 3.
TRAM flap utilizing periareolar incision with lateral extension before and after surgery.

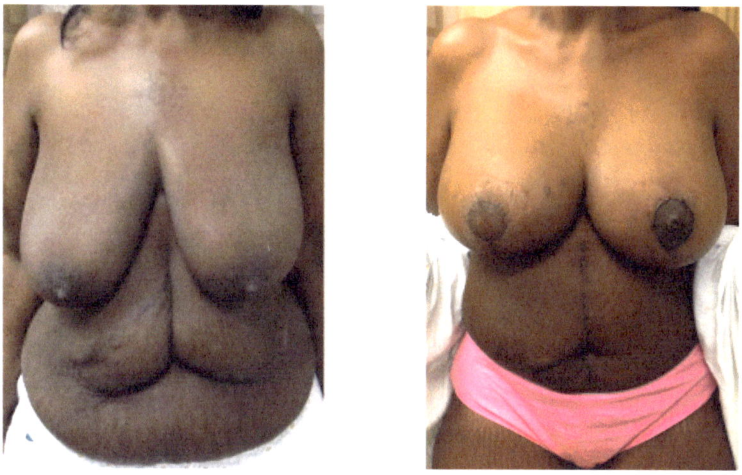

Figure 4.
TRAM flap utilizing wise pattern incision before and after surgery.

incisions that can be used with the aid of a plastic surgeon is a wise (**Figure 4**) or vertical pattern, similar to breast reduction or mastopexy incisions. These incisions allow for removal of excess skin that can be seen in ptotic patients. Additional benefits include reshaping of the breast mound and to allow for a smaller skin envelope for patients that desire a reduction in breast size.

With advances in breast cancer treatment the ability to preserve the nipple areolar complex is now possible. This not only allows for improved cosmesis but also quality of life for patients. The ideal patient for preservation of the nipple areolar complex would have a small breast, minimal ptosis (<grade 2), non-obese (BMI < 30 kg/m^2), and be a non-smoker [15]. There are techniques that will be described later in the chapter to allow for nipple areolar preservation in larger ptotic patients. From a cancer standpoint, patients that have NAC involvement seen on MRI, inflammatory breast cancer, extensive skin involvement, or bloody nipple discharge are not candidates for nipple sparing mastectomies [16].

5. Flaps

Free tissue transfers from an abdominal donor site is most commonly used for breast reconstruction. The TRAM, DIEP, and SIEA flaps all result in similar abdominal donor scars and include the lower abdominal skin/subcutaneous tissue between the umbilicus and the pubis in the flap. The deep inferior epigastric artery supplies the TRAM and DIEP flaps so various amounts of fascia, muscle, and nerve preservation is performed to allow for perforator harvest. In contrary, the SIEA flap is based on the superficial inferior epigastric artery so fascial violation does not occur. The majority of patients have small or absent superficial systems so SIEA flaps are only performed in a minority of patients [8].

An algorithm was developed by Lindsey in 2007 based on perforator anatomy to aid in selection of the appropriate abdominal flap [7]. Evaluation of the lateral row perforators proceeds the medial row perforators. If a large (>3 mm) centrally located perforator is seen from the deep inferior epigastric artery, then a single perforator DIEP can be performed. If moderate (1.5–3 mm) perforators are present, then more than one perforator should be included in the DIEP. When small (<1.5 mm) perforators are present then evaluation of the medial row perforators should be performed.

If the medial row perforators are also small (<1.5 mm) then a muscle sparing (MS) TRAM should be selected [7]. An SIEA flap can be considered if the vessel is large (>1.5 mm) and palpable but should be limited to smaller flaps [6].

If the abdomen is not available to use as a donor site then the thigh and gluteal areas can be used but require more difficult positioning in the operating room and the flaps tend to be smaller in size compared to abdominally based flaps.

5.1 Transverse rectus abdominis myocutaneous (TRAM)

The first abdominally based free and pedicled flaps for breast reconstruction were performed by Hartrampf and Holmstrom nearly 4 decades ago [4, 17]. To minimize donor site morbidity and vascular complications combined with the refinements in microsurgical technique, the free TRAM increased in popularity among surgeons. Even though the TRAM flap is a Mathes and Nahai type III muscle (two dominant vessels), it has a more robust blood supply based on the deep inferior epigastric artery compared to the internal thoracic artery [18]. The free TRAM is now the flap of choice for breast reconstruction in the majority of breast centers.

The TRAM flaps can spare various amounts of muscle to minimize abdominal wall morbidity so a classification system was developed by Nahabedian in 2002. A MS-0 TRAM involves the full width of the rectus abdominis muscle, MS-1 preserves the lateral or medial segment of muscle, MS-2 preserves the lateral and medial segment of muscle, and MS-3 (DIEP) preserves the entire muscle [19].

5.1.1 Marking

For any breast reconstruction patient, the markings for the breast should be in the standing position. The midline (sternal notch to pubis), inframammary folds (IMFs), anterior axillary lines, and the breast footprints are marked (**Figure 5**). If one of the IMF's are not apparent then the contralateral IMF can be used as a guide. A mastopexy incision marking can also be performed as needed. In a patient with a unilateral reconstruction, a symmetry procedure can be performed on the

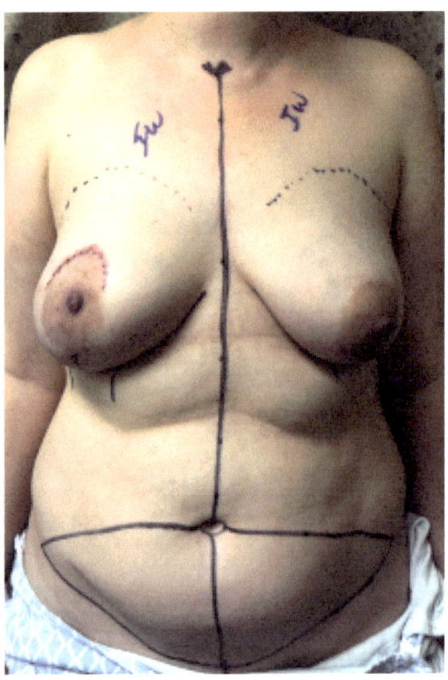

Figure 5.
TRAM/DIEP/SIEA flap markings.

contralateral side, which should also be marked at this time. It is important to put the nipple-areolar complex on the symmetry side to match the reconstructed breast and not at the level of the native IMF, as is done in routine breast reductions.

For the abdominal marking, the patient is in standing position to identify and mark the lower abdominal fold, which will hide the placement of the incision. In the midline, this incision should be at least 6 cm from the vulvar commissure to prevent urinary stream dysfunction post-operatively. The lower incision is typically extended laterally distal to the anterior superior iliac spine (ASIS) to remove any Burow's triangles. The upper incision is marked about the level of the umbilicus and then extended laterally to meet the lower incision endpoint (**Figure 5**). A pinch test must be used to confirm the location of the upper incision mark to ensure proper abdominal wall closure at the end of the case. It is also helpful to keep the length of the upper and lower incision limbs a similar length to prevent scalloping of the incision upon skin closure.

5.1.2 Flap dissection

The lower skin incision is made first followed by dissection of the SIEA/SIEV for a few centimeters to allow for superficial vascular supply as needed. The SIEA/SIEV can then be clipped and divided if they are not to be used for a SIEA flap. Dissection then proceeds all the way down to the muscular fascia but care should be taken to leave some fat around the ASIS to prevent injury to the lateral femoral cutaneous nerve, which is medial to the ASIS. After confirming the upper incision mark with a pinch test the upper incision can be made, including release of the umbilicus. The upper incision is taken down to the muscular fascia. The upper abdominal flap is then elevated above the muscular fascia in the midline to the xiphoid and costal margins as needed to aid in abdominal wall closure.

The dissection then continues from lateral to medial above the level of the muscular fascia until the lateral row perforators are encountered going through the anterior rectus fascia and into the flap (**Figure 6**). It is imperative to turn down the bovie or bipolar once you start to dissect the perforators. If a bilateral reconstruction is being performed, then the vertical midline incision can be made to separate the two flaps (**Figure 7**). Dissection then proceeds from medial to lateral above the level of the muscular fascia until the medial row perforators are encountered. If a unilateral reconstruction is being performed, then the vertical midline incision is

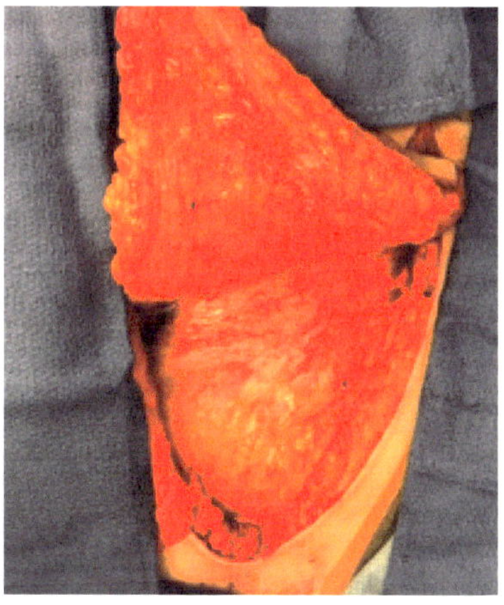

Figure 6.
Lateral to medial dissection of TRAM flap above muscular fascia to lateral row perforators.

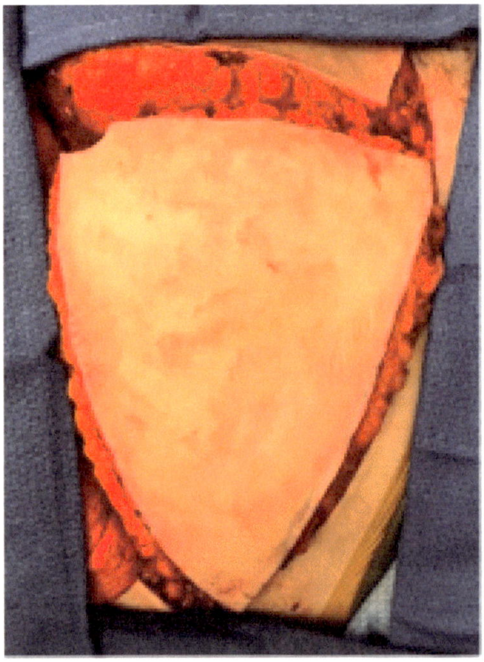

Figure 7.
Vertical midline incision separating bilateral TRAM flaps.

not performed. Dissection in this case then proceeds in the midline at the level of the muscular fascia until the medial row perforators are visualized. After visual inspection of all perforators, a Doppler can be used to see which perforators are more dominant. A decision is made (based on the above algorithm) about taking the lateral, medial, or both row perforators. Further dissection between the perforators along the muscular fascia occurs to help preserve fascia for the abdominal wall closure. A marking pen is used to design the planned longitudinal incision in the anterior rectus sheath, which is then extended to the lateral edge of the rectus inferiorly to aid in pedicle dissection. Various amount of anterior rectus sheath are incorporated into the flap depending on the number and location of the perforators. The anterior rectus sheath is incised and the lateral aspect of the sheath elevated off of the rectus abdominis muscle (**Figure 8**). The deep inferior epigastric artery/vein is then identified deep and lateral to the rectus abdominis muscle. The pedicle is then dissected all the way to the external iliac vessels and then separated near their origins (**Figure 9**). The pedicle is then dissected superiorly to identify the perforators going into the flap. Care should be taken to preserve the vascular and nerve supply to the rectus abdominis muscle. The rectus abdominis muscle is then split longitudinally between the perforators and the rectus abdominis muscle that will remain in-situ (**Figure 10**). If a MS-2 TRAM is being performed then a second longitudinal spit is made in the rectus abdominis muscle on the other side of the perforators. Once the pedicle is cleared posteriorly from the posterior rectus sheath, then the pedicle can be dissected away from the rectus abdominis muscle inferior to the takeoff of the first perforator. The rectus abdominis muscle can then be divided with cautery inferiorly with care taken to protect the pedicle. Attention is then turned to identify the superior epigastric vessels, which are then temporarily clamped. The Doppler is used to identify perforators on the skin, which can then be marked with a 5-0 prolene suture. After confirming the vascular supply to the flap, the superior rectus abdominis muscle and the superior epigastric vessels can be divided (**Figure 11**). The deep inferior epigastric vessels should not be divided until the recipient vessels are identified.

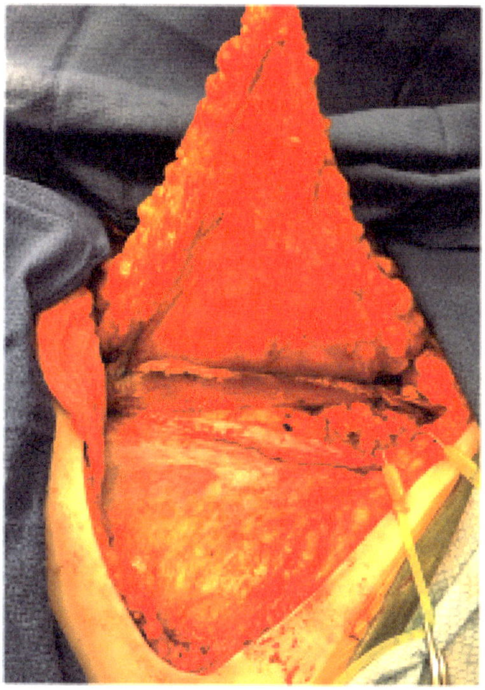

Figure 8.
Lateral anterior rectus sheath elevated after fascial incision.

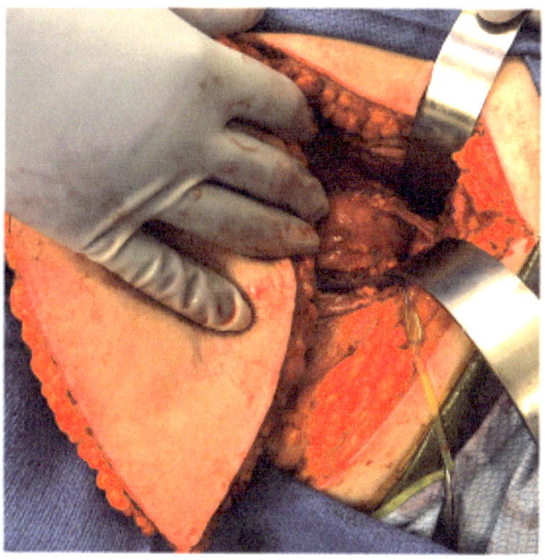

Figure 9.
TRAM flap pedicle dissection to external iliac vessels.

5.1.3 Recipient vessel harvest

After completion of the mastectomy attention is then turned to the chest to harvest recipient vessels, typically the internal mammary vessels or the thoracodorsal vessels. The internal mammary vessels at our institution are preferred because the thoracodorsal vessels can be damaged during the mastectomy or lymph node dissection and require a long pedicle to allow for medialization of the flap. Some prefer the thoracodorsal vessels because of easier dissection but either recipient vessel has the same outcomes and are proven to be safe and reliable [20].

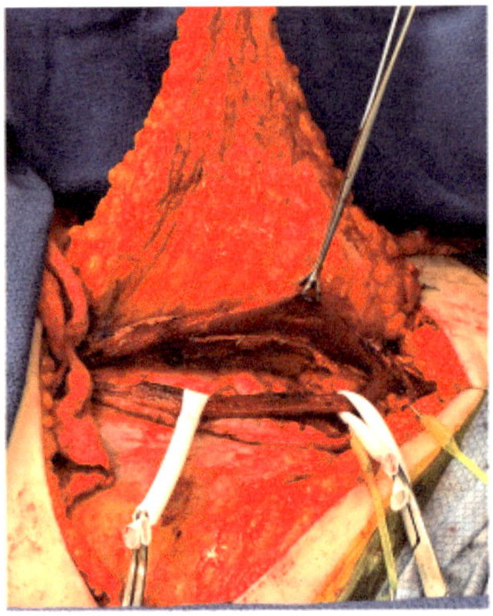

Figure 10.
TRAM flap after longitudinal split of rectus muscle with exposed pedicle.

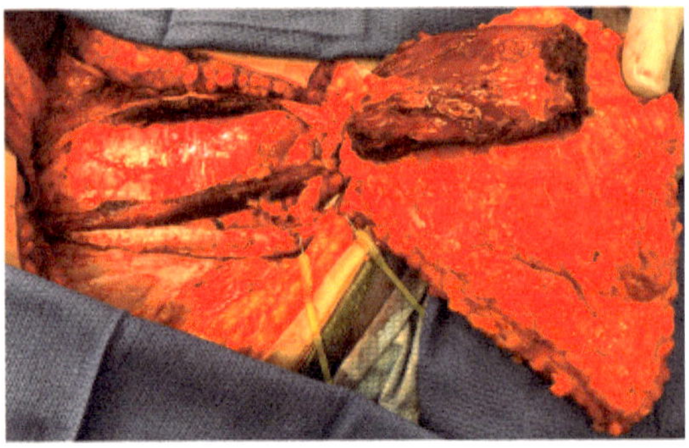

Figure 11.
TRAM flap in-situ after division of rectus muscle.

To expose the internal mammary vessels, the mastectomy skin is gently retracted and then the pectoralis major muscle is split over the third costal cartilage. A Weitlaner retractor is placed between the split pectoralis major muscle for exposure. The third costal cartilage perichondrium is incised anteriorly from the sternal attachment then 2–3 cm laterally. A freer elevator is used to elevate the perichondrium anteriorly then posteriorly off of the third costal cartilage. The third costal cartilage segment can be incised sharply laterally with use of a Doyen rib raspatory to protect the pleura posteriorly. The third costal cartilage is then removed in piecemeal fashion using a rongeur until the sternal edge is encountered. Some prefer not to use the Doyen rib raspatory and only use the rongeur. Bipolar is then used to remove the third costal cartilage perichondrium along with some of the adjacent intercostal muscles. As the internal mammary vessels are encountered about 1 cm lateral to the sternal edge, it is important to clip any small branches from the vessels entering the posterior perichondrium. Care is taken to preserve the anterior branch of the third intercostal nerve if flap re-innervation is desired. The internal mammary vessels can be dissected as needed to obtain length. If one is struggling with the vessels dissection it is important to finish further dissection with increased loupe magnification or the microscope. An internal mammary lymph node is often encountered along the artery, which can be sent for permanent pathology to aid in oncologic staging. A neurosurgical patty and microsurgery background sheet is

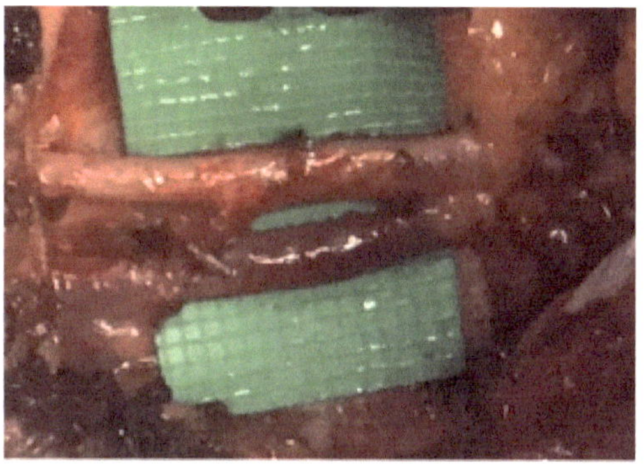

Figure 12.
Internal mammary vessel preparation.

then placed posterior to the internal mammary vessels (**Figure 12**). Vasodilating agents such as lidocaine 4% or papaverine can be injected around the vessels per surgeon preference and then covered with a warm moist RayTec sponge. The retraction on the mastectomy flaps should be released to allow for improved perfusion until the microsurgical anastomosis will be performed.

For exposure of the thoracodorsal vessels, the mastectomy skin is gently retracted to allow for visualization of the anterior border of the latissimus dorsi muscle. Once identified, the anterior border of the latissimus dorsi muscle is followed superiorly to the axillary vein. The thoracodorsal vessels will then be located between the chest wall and the latissimus dorsi muscle. The vessels are dissected until the appropriate length and caliber is obtained. Another option for recipient vessels that are less commonly used are the thoracoacromial vessels. These vessels are identified in the midclavicular area by using a Doppler. The pectoralis major muscle is then split and dissection of the thoracoacromial vessels occurs. The axillary vessels and the scapular circumflex vessels can also be used if the above recipient sites are not available. Additional venous drainage can occur via cephalic vein or external jugular vein transposition [21].

5.1.4 Anastomosis

Once the recipient vessels are dissected and the TRAM flap elevated, the flap pedicle can be clipped and divided. The artery should be clipped prior to the vein so the flap does not get engorged with blood. The flap is placed on an iced lap sponge and then transferred to the contralateral chest. The flap is rotated 90° so the pedicle lies adjacent to the recipient vessels. Care is taken to make sure the flap pedicle is laying in its natural orientation without twisting. The flap is secured to the chest wall using sutures and/or staples. A microscope is then brought into the field if loupe magnification is not preferred and centered over the recipient vessels. The pedicle vessels are further dissected until enough length is obtained and the vessel ends are cleared of fat and adventitia. Attention is then turned to the recipient vessels, which are dissected in a similar fashion. An Acland clamp is placed proximally on the recipient artery and vein and then the distal ends clipped and divided. The recipient vessels should be irrigated with heparinized saline (100 units per ml) until the lumen is clear. The flap should also be flushed with heparinized saline through the artery until the venous output is clear. After the recipient and pedicle vessels are prepared, the vessels ends are approximated in a way to ensure no kinking or twisting of the vessels. The first anastomosis performed is the vessel which will be more posterior after the artery and venous anastomoses are completed. For the

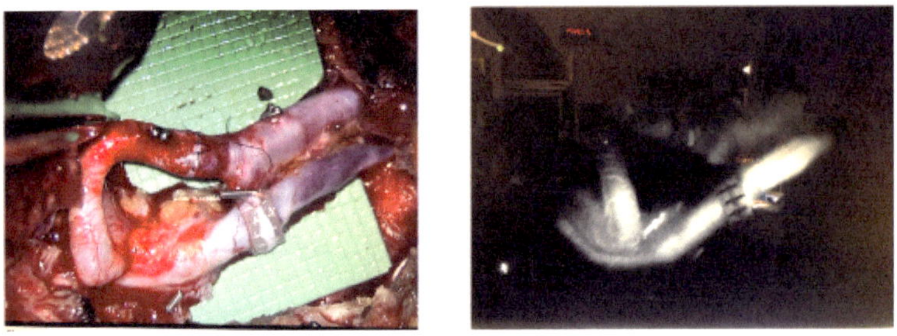

Figure 13.
Internal mammary vessel anastomosis and ICG angiography.

artery, the double apposing Acland clamp can be used to approximate the arterial ends if needed. 8-0 or 9-0 nylon is used in an interrupted fashion for the arterial anastomosis. The venous anastomosis is performed using a venous coupler after the diameters of the veins are measured. The use of the venous coupler has been shown to reduce operating room times and take-backs to the operating room [22]. The venous followed by the arterial Acland clamps are released and the vessels checked for leakage and patency. We routinely use indocyanine green angiography to evaluate anastomotic patency [23, 24] (**Figure 13**). A study by Holm showed that the intrinsic transit time (ITT) or the time it takes for the indocyanine green dye to travel from the arterial to the venous anastomosis can help predict flap compromise and early re-exploration. An ITT greater than 50 s was significantly associated with these negative outcomes [24].

5.2 Deep inferior epigastric perforator (DIEP)

As techniques in microsurgery developed along with the need to reduce the amount of donor muscle sacrifice, the DIEP flap was developed and first performed by Allen in 1994 [5]. Some consider the DIEP flap the gold standard for autologous breast reconstruction but there can be higher fat necrosis rates compared to the TRAM flap if only a few perforators are included in the flap [6].

Similar to the TRAM flap, the DIEP flap can preserve various amounts of muscle and nerves. Based on the Nahabedian classification, DIEP flaps are considered MS-3 TRAM flaps because they preserve the entire rectus muscle [19]. Lee in 2010 developed a DIEP classification because not all DIEP flap harvests are the same as they vary with how much muscle and nerves are transected. A DIEP-1 has one perforator and preserves all muscle and nerves. A DIEP-2 has two or more perforators in the same row requiring segmental nerve sacrifice but the muscle is preserved. A DIEP-3 has perforators in different rows so both muscle and nerve are sacrificed. When comparing the DIEP-1 to DIEP-3 flaps, the DIEP-1 flaps had a significantly higher fat necrosis rate (19.8 vs. 9.2%) [6].

5.2.1 Flap dissection

The breast and abdomen markings pre-operatively are the same as for the TRAM flap above (**Figure 5**). The lower and upper abdominal incisions are made with dissection/preservation of the superficial inferior epigastric vessels. The lateral and medial row perforators are identified in standard fashion. The surgeon then determines which perforators to include in the flap. A DIEP-1 can be performed if the perforator is greater than 3 mm. If the perforators are between 1.5 and 3 mm, a DIEP-2 or DIEP 3 can be performed. However, if no perforators are greater than 1.5 mm, a TRAM should be considered [6, 7]. Usually if there are multiple

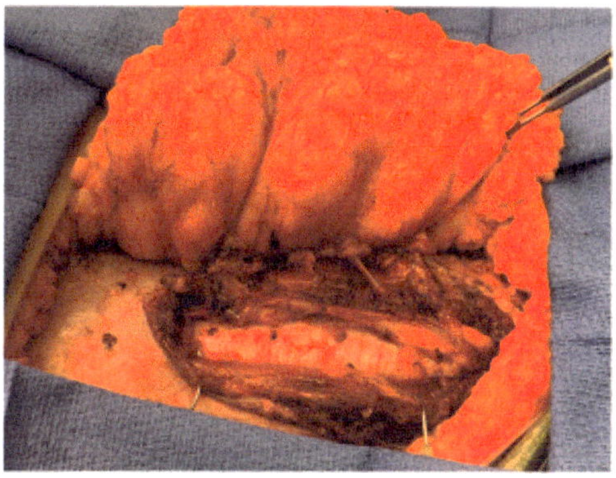

Figure 14.
Longitudinal rectus muscle longitudinal split during DIEP flap harvest.

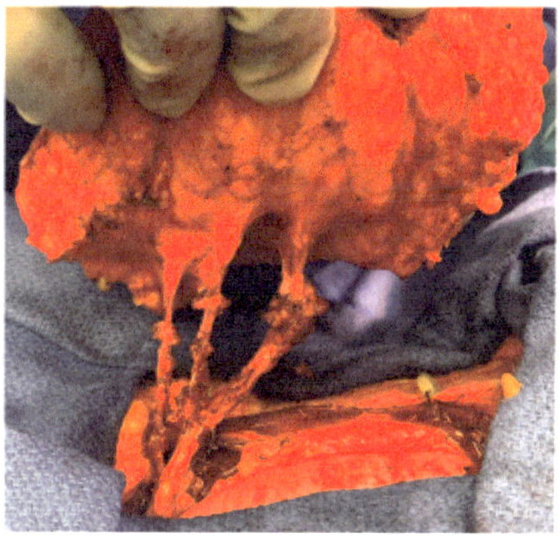

Figure 15.
DIEP flap based on three perforators.

perforators in the same row, they will all be included in the DIEP flap. In order to preserve more fascia and muscle dissection certain perforators can be temporarily clamped so the flap can be assessed based on desired perforators. The ideal perforators should not only be large but also centrally located to allow for centric perfusion. Once the perforators are selected the anterior rectus sheath is incised, the pedicle identified, and the rectus muscle split longitudinally adjacent to the perforators (**Figure 14**). The perforators are dissected circumferentially from the pedicle to the fascia. A small fascial cuff around the perforators can be left intact if the perforators are tiny or if the surgeons prefers. Once the perforators and pedicle are dissected, the flap should be assessed for perfusion after the extraneous perforators and superior epigastric vessels are temporarily clamped. The extraneous perforators and superior epigastric vessels can then be clipped and divided (**Figure 15**). In a unilateral reconstruction, the contralateral perforators should be left intact as a backup if needed. Once the recipient vessels are prepared the DIEP flap pedicle can be clipped and divided (**Figure 16**).

5.3 Superficial inferior epigastric artery (SIEA)

In 1991, Grotting was the first person to use a free SIEA flap for breast reconstruction [25]. Compared to the TRAM and DIEP flaps, the SIEA flap minimizes donor site morbidity because it does not violate the rectus fascia. Therefore, the risks

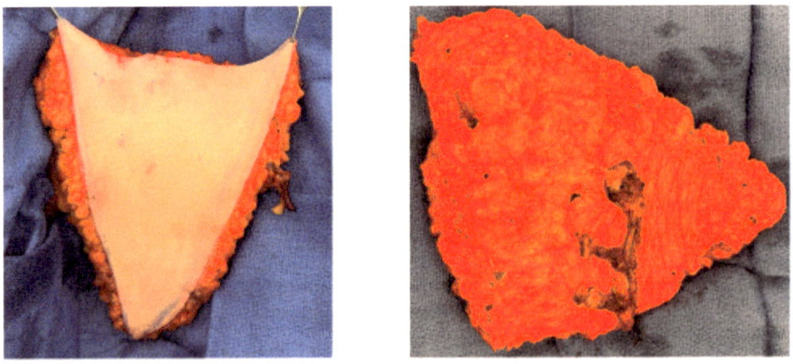

Figure 16.
Anterior and posterior surfaces of the DIEP flap with visible superficial inferior epigastric vein.

of hernia, bulging, and abdominal wall weakness are reduced. Other benefits of the SIEA flap is that it can reduce patient discomfort and hospital stay [8]. The SIEA flap is performed in the minority of patients because 35–51% of patients do not have an SIEA [8, 26]. Other disadvantages of the SIEA flap is it can only perfuse zones I and II, has a short pedicle length (5–8 cm), and the pedicle exits the flap just below the skin. The use of the SIEA flap should be performed if the vessel is palpable with a diameter that is at least 1.5 mm [8, 27]. If the SIEA is absent or small then one should proceed to evaluating the deep inferior epigastric perforators as discussed above.

5.3.1 Flap dissection

The breast and abdomen markings for the SIEA flap is the same as the TRAM and DIEP flaps (**Figure 5**). The lower abdominal incision is made and then the SIEA is identified. The SIEA is usually one third of the distance from the pubic tubercle to the ASIS. A couple techniques to help identify the SIEA is the use of Doppler or to apply traction on both sides of the lower incision with your fingers to help separate the fat from the SIEA. The SIEA and SIEV can be dissected to their origin on the superficial circumflex iliac vessels or less commonly the femoral vessels. If one is not confident that the SIEA will perfuse the flap, the deep inferior epigastric perforators can be dissected suprafascial and then temporarily clamped so the perfusion of the flap can be assessed. Once perfusion of the flap is confirmed, then the deep perforators can be transected and the pedicle clipped/divided. The flap needs to be placed medially to allow the short pedicle to reach the internal mammary vessels. Hence, the ipsilateral SIEA flap is preferred.

5.4 Transverse upper gracilis (TUG)

For patients that have contraindications to using abdominal tissue for breast reconstruction or who do not want a scar from hip to hip they can use their thigh tissue. Another benefit of using thigh tissue as a donor site is that it can result in a thigh lift and the scar is usually inconspicuous. The transverse upper gracilis (TUG) flap was modified by Yousif in 1992 to allow for improved skin paddle survival [28]. It was not until 2002 when Arnez performed the first free TUG flap for breast reconstruction [29].

The TUG flap is a Mathes and Nahai type II flap with the dominant vascular supply from the ascending branch of the medial circumflex femoral artery [18]. The pedicle is around 6 cm in length and enters the gracilis muscle on its medial side about 8–10 cm inferior to the pubic tubercle [29, 30]. There are one or two minor pedicles from the superficial femoral artery that enter the distal aspect of the gracilis muscle [29].

5.4.1 Marking

The breast markings are performed in the standard fashion (**Figure 5**). The patient is then frogged legged with the thigh abducted and externally rotated. The adductor longus is marked from the pubis to the medial femoral condyle. The gracilis muscle is located 2–3 cm posterior to this line. A doppler is used to identity the perforator for the TUG flap 8–10 cm inferior to the pubic tubercle over the gracilis muscle. The skin paddle is centered over the perforator and the vertical height of the flap determined by a pinch test (**Figure 17**). Primary closure can occur with a width of 10–12 cm. The proximal incision marking is at or 1 fingerbreadth below the groin crease and extends from just lateral to the adductor longus to the midline of the posterior thigh along the gluteal crease. The distal incision marking is then drawn to form a semilunar skin paddle that can have a length up to 25 cm [31, 32].

5.4.2 Flap dissection

The patient is placed in the supine position with the thigh abducted and the knee flexed. The anterior part of the flap is raised first above the level of the muscular fascia. Care is taken to preserve the saphenous vein but the posterior branch can be included in the flap. Once the medial aspect of the adductor longus is reached, the muscular fascia is incised. The interval between the adductor longus and gracilis is entered so the pedicle can be identified entering the medial aspect of the gracilis muscle. The ascending branch of the medial circumflex femoral artery is dissected all the way to the profunda femoris artery, which can allow for a pedicle length of 5–6 cm [29, 31]. After the pedicle is dissected, the posterior aspect of the flap can be raised above the muscular fascia. At the posterior aspect of the gracilis, the dissection becomes subfascial. The gracilis muscle is then transected 3 cm above and below the entrance of the pedicle. The obturator nerve branch to the gracilis is clipped and divided followed by the pedicle. In contrast to the abdominal flaps, the TUG flap needs to be coned by approximating the superior edges of the two wings

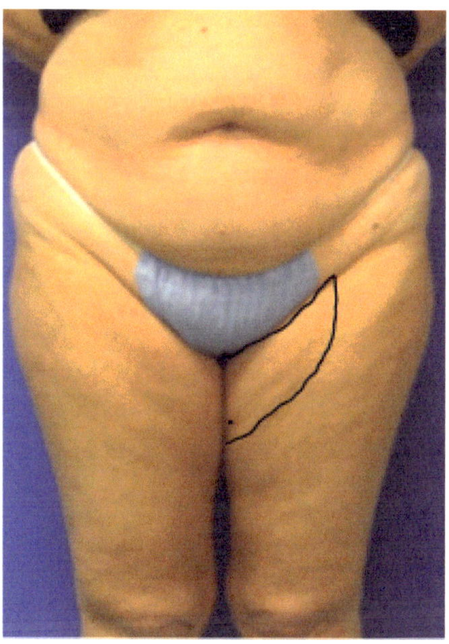

Figure 17.
TUG flap and perforator markings.

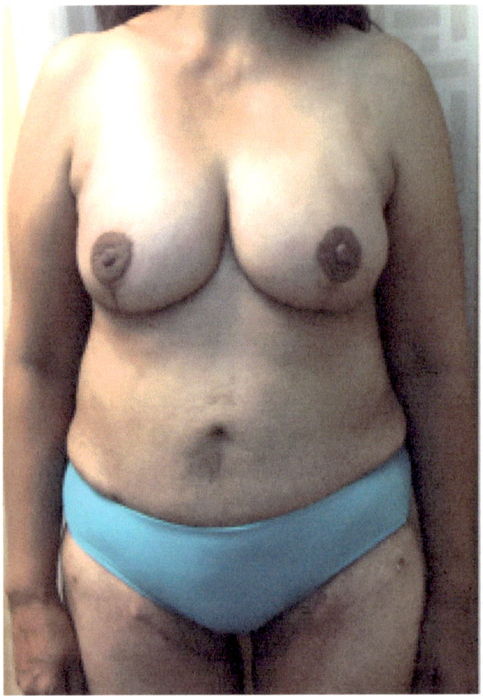

Figure 18.
Bilateral breast reconstruction using TUG flaps.

of the flap. The apex of the coned flap can then be used to reconstruct a nipple areolar complex (NAC). The post-operative results of a patient that underwent bilateral TUG flaps for breast reconstruction is shown in **Figure 18**.

5.5 Profunda artery perforator (PAP)

Another thigh-based flap for patients with contraindications to abdominal donor tissue is the profunda artery perforator (PAP) flap, which was first performed by Allen and Haddock in 2010 for breast reconstruction [33, 34]. Prior to this in 2000, Angrigiani developed the PAP flap based on the first medial branch of the profunda femoris artery [35]. Suitable patients for a PAP flap would have excess tissue in the posterior medial thigh and small to moderate sized breasts [34].

The PAP flap is a fasciocutaneous flap that is based on the second or third perforator from the profunda femoris artery. The pedicle length can be up to 13 cm and can be septocutaneous or go through the adductor magnus muscle [36]. The benefits of the PAP flap over the TUG flap is it has a larger volume, longer pedicle, requires no muscle sacrifice, and less anterior thigh scar. The PAP flap can also be converted to a TUG or IGAP flap if needed intra-operatively [36].

5.5.1 Marking

The breast markings are made in standard fashion (**Figure 5**) then the patient is placed in the supine position with the thigh abducted and knee flexed. The gracilis muscle is identified just posterior to the adductor longus muscle. A mark is made 2 cm posterior to the gracilis muscle and 8 cm inferior to the groin crease. A Doppler is used to confirm the perforator around this location [35]. There are also other posterior or lateral thigh perforators from the profunda femoris artery that

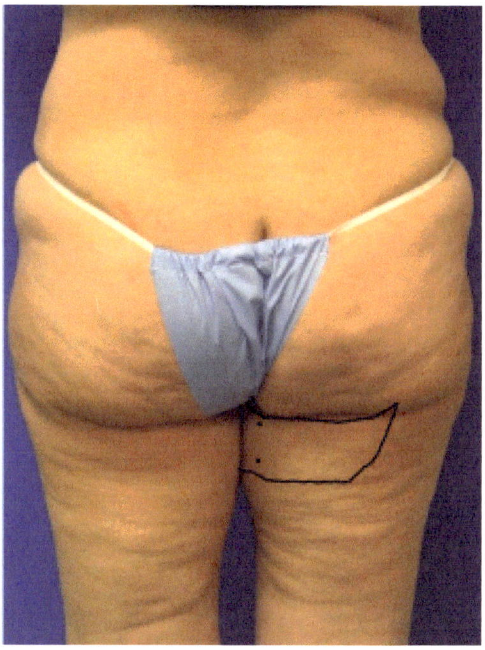

Figure 19.
PAP flap and perforator markings.

are seen on preoperative CTA or MRA that can be used but the medial perforators are preferred because of ease of positioning and size of the medial perforators [34]. The flap is designed in an ellipse shape with the superior border of the flap at or 1 cm below the gluteal crease and the inferior border around 7 cm below the superior marking (**Figure 19**). A pinch test can also be performed to increase the vertical height of the flap if needed. Care is taken to make sure the flap is centered on the marked perforator(s). The length of the flap can be up to 35 cm, which extends from the posterior lateral thigh to the medial thigh. If the TUG flap is being considered as a bailout plan then the medial incision should be carried to the adductor longus [37]. If more posterior perforators are being considered the patient can be in the prone position.

5.5.2 Flap dissection

Similar to the TUG flap, the PAP flap is performed in the supine position with the thigh abducted and knee flexed. The anterior medial aspect of the flap is raised above the level of the muscular fascia until the posterior border of the adductor longus is reached. A subfascial plane is dissected between the adductor longus and gracilis muscles. The perforator to the PAP flap can be identified along the adductor magnus muscle as you dissect posteriorly. If no perforator is seen then the flap can be converted to a TUG flap. After confirming the perforator to the PAP flap the gracilis muscle can be retracted anteriorly to aid in further perforator dissection. If further pedicle length is needed then the pedicle can be dissected to the profunda femoris artery (**Figure 20**). The posterior lateral aspect of the flap can then be dissected in the suprafascial plane and then below the fascia once the perforator is nearby. To increase volume in the flap and improve lateral thigh contour, the flap can be beveled in the lateral thigh [34]. The pedicle to the flap can be clipped and divided after the flap is elevated. The PAP flap is coned in the same fashion as the TUG flap with the apex of the flap able to reconstruct the NAC as needed.

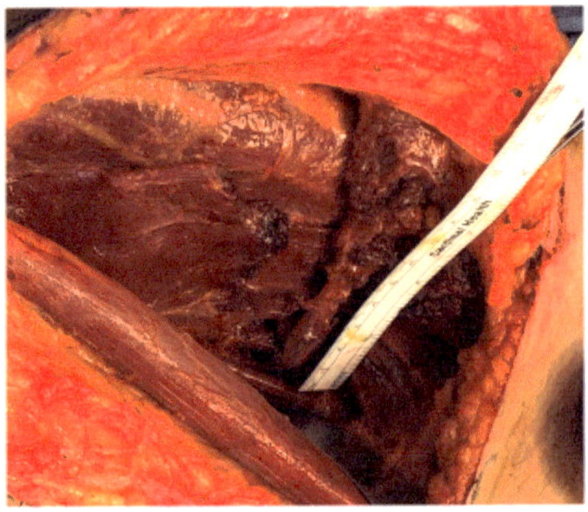

Figure 20.
PAP flap pedicle dissected through adductor magnus muscle to the profunda femoris artery.

5.6 Superior gluteal artery perforator (SGAP)

Breast reconstruction can be performed by utilizing gluteal tissue if the abdomen and thighs are not usable as donor sites. The first superior gluteal artery myocutaneous flap for breast reconstruction was by Fujino in 1975 [38]. With the development of perforator flaps, Allen in 1993 developed the superior gluteal artery perforator (SGAP) flap to allow for a longer vascular pedicle and gluteus maximus muscle preservation [39, 40]. The use of the SGAP is not considered the first option for breast reconstruction because of a tedious flap dissection, change in positioning in the operating room, smaller volume flap, and gluteal scarring [40].

The SGAP flap is based on the superior gluteal artery, which is a branch of the internal iliac artery. The superior gluteal artery leaves the pelvis above the piriformis muscle and then divides into a deep and superficial branch. The superficial branch transverses the gluteal muscles and gives off perforators to the skin [30]. The use of CTA or MRA preoperatively can be used to aid in identification of the SGAP perforators.

5.6.1 Marking

To aid in intra-operative positioning, the patient is placed in the lateral decubitus position and the ipsilateral flap is used so a two team approach can be utilized for the chest and gluteal areas. If bilateral gluteal flaps are needed then the patient will have to be in the prone position for flap harvest after the mastectomies and recipient vessels are harvested. The posterior superior iliac spine (PSIS), anterior superior iliac spine (ASIS), greater trochanter, and coccyx are marked. The perforators are identified one third of the distance from the PSIS to the greater trochanter, which is confirmed with Doppler. There can be more lateral perforators located between the gluteus maximus and gluteus medius muscles that can allow for a longer pedicle length, which can be included in the flap. The flap is then centered on a line from the coccyx to the ASIS. It is desirable to have a less centric but more laterally placed perforator, which will allow for a longer pedicle. The height of the flap can vary from 7 to 14 cm but must be confirmed with the pinch test to allow for appropriate closure (**Figure 21**). The length of the flap can also vary from 18 to 30 cm [30, 40].

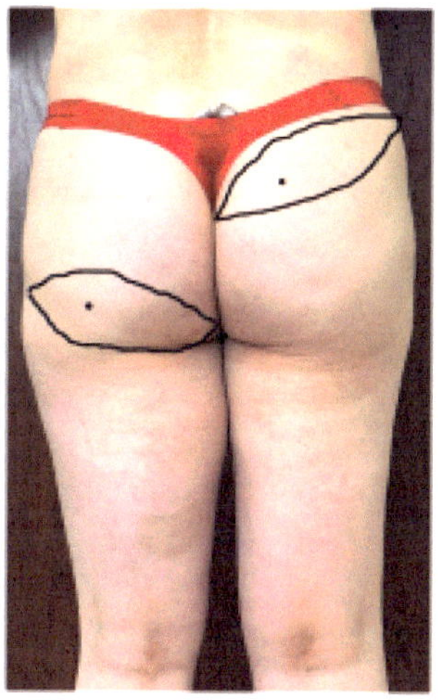

Figure 21.
SGAP (right) and IGAP (left) flap and perforator markings.

5.6.2 Flap dissection

The SGAP flap skin incisions are made and then beveled outward once past the superficial fascia to increase flap volume and to improve the transition onto the chest wall. The gluteus maximus fascia is incised and then the dissection proceeds in this plane above the muscle from lateral to medial until the perforators are identified. Similar to DIEP flap dissection, the dominant perforators are identified and preserved. Usually one large perforator is selected but two perforators in the same muscle fiber plane can also be dissected together. The selected perforators are dissected vertically between the gluteus maximus muscle fibers and through the deep gluteal fascia until a fat pad is seen. Once the pedicle is of the appropriate size and length the dissection can cease. In a unilateral reconstruction in the lateral decubitus position, the pedicle to the flap can be clipped and divided followed by the microvascular anastomoses. If a bilateral reconstruction is performed in the prone position, the flaps should be placed in a bag on an ice saline bath. The patient is then flipped supine so the anastomoses can be performed. The internal mammary vessels are the main recipient vessels for the SGAP flap. If the SGAP flap has two perforators then one can be connected in an antegrade fashion and the other in a retrograde fashion to the internal mammary vessels. After confirming flap perfusion, the flap can be coned or the tips excised to improve flap contour [30, 40].

5.7 Inferior gluteal artery perforator (IGAP)

The inferior gluteal artery perforator (IGAP) flap is another gluteal based free flap for breast reconstruction. The first IGAP free flap for breast reconstruction was performed by LeQuang in 1978 [41]. The ideal patient will have excess tissue in the inferior buttock or a saddlebag deformity. The benefit of the IGAP flap over the SGAP flap is the scar can be hidden in the gluteal crease and it does not leave a hollowing in the superior gluteal area [42]. However, the IGAP flap tends to be smaller than the SGAP and can lead to increased patient discomfort if the sciatic nerve is exposed [27].

The IGAP flap is based on the inferior gluteal artery, which is a branch of the internal iliac artery. The inferior gluteal artery leaves the pelvis below the piriformis muscle and is soon accompanied by the sciatic nerve, posterior femoral cutaneous nerve, and the internal pudendal vessels [32]. The IGAP can also be neurotized if the inferior gluteal nerve is preserved. Similar to other perforator flaps, preoperative CTA or MRA can be used to aid in identification of the IGAP perforators.

5.7.1 Marking

The gluteal crease is marked in the standing position. The positioning of the patient for the IGAP flap is the same as for the SGAP flap. Lateral decubitus for a unilateral reconstruction and prone for a bilateral reconstruction. The PSIS and ischial tuberosity are marked. The inferior gluteal perforators are identified two third of the distance from the PSIS to the outer aspect of the ischial tuberosity. The inferior border of the flap is marked at or 1 cm inferior to the gluteal crease. After confirming the location of the IGAP perforators with a doppler, the superior border of the flap is marked to form an ellipse that is parallel to the gluteal crease [42]. The height of the flap is usually around 7–8 cm but must be confirmed with a pinch test (**Figure 21**). The length of the flap is around 18 cm. The flap can be designed to include the saddle bag deformity laterally. Care must be taken to leave tissue over the ischial tuberosity to prevent patient discomfort and wound dehiscence when in the sitting position [30].

5.7.2 Flap dissection

The IGAP flap skin incisions are made and then continued just distal to the gluteus maximus fascia. Beveling of the flap can occur to increase flap volume or to remove tissue in the saddle bag area. The dissection proceeds in this plane above the muscle from lateral to medial until the inferior gluteal artery perforators are identified. Typically, two to four perforators from the inferior gluteal artery can be identified but the dominant perforators are preserved [42]. Usually one perforator that is greater than 1 mm is selected but two perforators in the same muscle fiber plane can also be dissected together. The selected perforators are dissected vertically between the gluteus maximus muscle fibers and through the deep gluteal fascia. Once the pedicle is of the appropriate size and length the dissection can cease. Similar to the SGAP harvest, a unilateral reconstruction in the lateral decubitus position can then proceed with pedicle clipping and dividing followed by the microvascular anastomoses. If a bilateral reconstruction is performed in the prone position, the flaps should be placed in a bag on an ice saline bath. The patient is then flipped supine so the anastomoses can be performed. The recipient vessels for the IGAP flap are the internal mammary vessels but they can also reach the thoracodorsal vessels since the pedicle length is around 8–11 cm. The elliptical IGAP flap is coned or the tips trimmed after the microvascular anastomoses [30, 42].

6. Insetting

After the arterial and venous anastomoses are deemed to be patent by using various techniques such as the strip test, uplift test, checking for dermal bleeding, and SPY-angiography, the flap should be placed into the breast pocket gently as to not avulse the anastomosis. If an abdominal flap is performed, the contralateral flap is usually chosen and rotated 90° so the corner of the flap with the umbilical carve out is placed inferior laterally. Therefore the vertical height of the flap will represent the width of the reconstructed breast. If the thoracodorsal vessels are preferred, then an ipsilateral flap should be used and rotated 90° so the pedicle vessels exit the flap laterally. A limitation to using the thoracodorsal vessels include the inability to medialize the flap that can result in a narrow breast. The rotation of the flaps can also be modified to increase or decrease the new breast mound width and/or height.

The shape of the neo-breast mound can be over looked and is a critical proponent to breast reconstruction from an esthetic standpoint. The first step to aid in shaping of the breast is to trim the flap to the desired breast footprint. Often it is necessary to trim and tapper the most lateral aspect of the flap or zone 4 to improve the contour of the upper pole of the breast. The projection of the flap can also be easily modified by folding the flap on itself or coning. In unilateral breast reconstructions, stacked or bipedicled abdominal free flap can be performed to increase volume as needed [43]. Once the shape of the flap is optimal, the flap should circumferentially be sutured down to the chest wall using 2-0 absorbable suture. Usually the medial aspect of the flap is sutured first to insure medial fullness of the neo-breast mound. The superficial fascia and/or dermis of the flap can be sutured to the deep fascia and inframammary fold (IMF) of the chest.

7. Mastectomy flap assessment and skin closure

Upon completion of flap in-setting, the viability of the mastectomy skin should be performed. Clear areas of devascularized mastectomy skin should be sharply excised. For areas of the mastectomy skin that are not so obvious, indocyanine green (ICG) angiography can be used to assess perfusion (**Figure 22**).

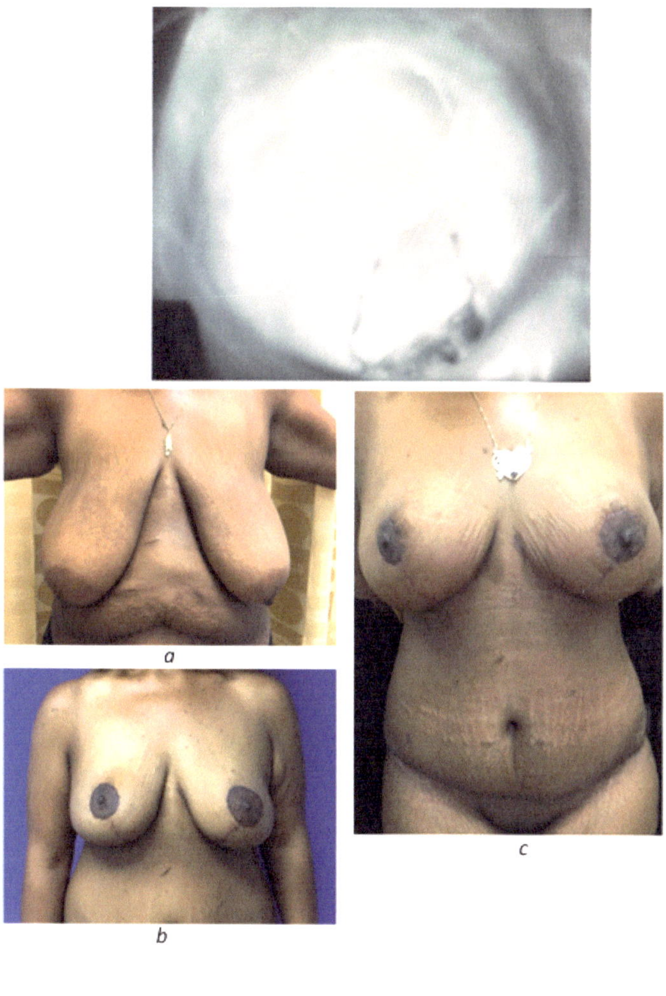

Figure 22.
Mastectomy skin, NAC, and flap perfusion assessment using ICG angiography. (a and b) First stage bilateral breast reduction before and after and (c) second stage bilateral NSM and TRAM flaps.

The trimming of mastectomy skin with the use of ICG imaging reduces the need for future operations secondary to deep skin necrosis [44]. Another alternative if a large or critical area of mastectomy skin is concerning for poor perfusion, the flap can be buried and then a second look procedure in 72 h can be performed to re-assess the mastectomy skin [45]. Aside from excising devascularized mastectomy skin, areas with significant radiation changes, scarring, and/or tethering need to be excised to allow for optimal outcomes. If the mastectomy skin is constricted causing pin cushioning of the flap, a superior lateral incision in the mastectomy skin can allow for release of the constricted mastectomy skin.

Once the mastectomy skin defect is known, the skin paddle on the flap can be designed. The excess skin on the outside of the skin paddle is then de-epithelialized using Gorney scissors or a scalpel. It is important to preserve the dermis in order to protect the subdermal plexus of the flap. However, from an esthetic standpoint to prevent an indentation along the flap suture line it is necessary to score the dermis about 1–2 mm away from the skin paddle. Prior to skin closure, hemostasis in the breast pocket and along the de-epithelized flap need to be confirmed. A 15F round channel drain is placed along the axilla and IMF then exits the skin inferior to the IMF along the anterior axillary line. The dermis is then approximated using 2-0 or 3-0 absorbable suture followed by 4-0 running subcuticular for the skin. The Doppler signal on the skin paddle should be confirmed and marked with a 5-0 prolene suture. Our preferred dressings for the flap incision is antibiotic ointment and xeroform then coverage with abdomen battle dressing (ABD) pads.

8. Ptosis management

Nipple-sparing mastectomy (NSM) has increased overtime with refinements in oncologic techniques and protocols, allowing for improved patient satisfaction and esthetics [46]. Patients with large or ptotic breasts were traditionally contraindicated to have nipple preservation over concerns of poor mastectomy skin and nipple perfusion. Some techniques that have been developed to increase nipple perfusion in ptotic patients include mastopexy or reduction (**Figure 22a–c**) before NSM, mastopexy during the time of the NSM, and nipple devascularization [47–49].

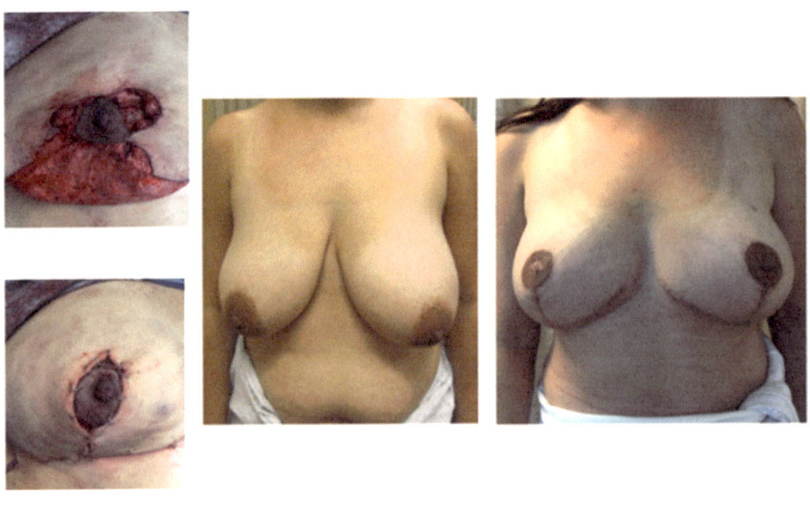

Figure 23.
Single stage bilateral NSM, de-epithelization wise pattern mastopexy, and TRAM flaps.

The use of mastectomy or reduction with a minimum of 3–4 weeks prior to nipple sparing mastectomy was performed by Spear in fifteen patients. No reports of total nipple-areola complex necrosis occurred and 13% had partial nipple-areola complex necrosis [47]. It is important to note that the majority of patients in this study underwent prophylactic NSM's because by adding an additional procedure can delay oncologic treatment of cancer patients. Another technique is to perform the mastopexy at the time of the nipple sparing mastectomy, which can be in a peri-areolar, vertical, or wise fashion [48]. Nguyen described an approach of skin reduction with deepithelization and tissue infolding that preserves dermal plexus perfusion and promotes nipple and skin flap survival in immediate breast reconstruction after skin sparing and NSM [49] (**Figure 23**).

Staged devascularization of the NAC can also be performed 1–3 weeks prior to NSM [50, 51]. This is performed by using a pre-existing incision or making a vertical or radial lateral incision then undermining the NAC and the adjacent skin for 4–5 cm in the mastectomy plane. During this time a biopsy of the subnipple is performed to confirm absence of tumor. The staged devascularization of the NAC in a study by Jensen in 20 patients resulted in 100% NAC survival after the NSM [50]. A follow up study by Nguyen a few years later also support the use of staged devascularization of the NAC in high risk women that undergo NSM [51, 52].

9. Adjunctive procedures

9.1 Neurotization

The ideal reconstructed breast should not only take into consideration size, shape, symmetry, and softness but also sensibility. The presence of sensation in the reconstructed breast has shown to improve patient satisfaction and quality of life [53]. The neurotization of abdominally based free tissue transfers have shown to have significantly increased sensory recovery [53, 54]. Coaptation of the flap nerve is typically performed to the anterior branch of the third intercostal nerve (**Figure 24**). This donor nerve can be found just below the third rib and crosses just anterior to the internal mammary vessels. The benefits of using the anterior branch of the third intercostal nerve is minimal dissection needed and it is in the vicinity of the vascular anastomoses. A less commonly used donor nerve is the lateral cutaneous branch of the third or fourth intercostal nerve because it can be damaged with the mastectomy procedure and is far away from the flap pedicle [54]. If primary coaptation of the nerves is not possible, a nerve conduit or graft can be used to improve sensibility. A meta-analysis

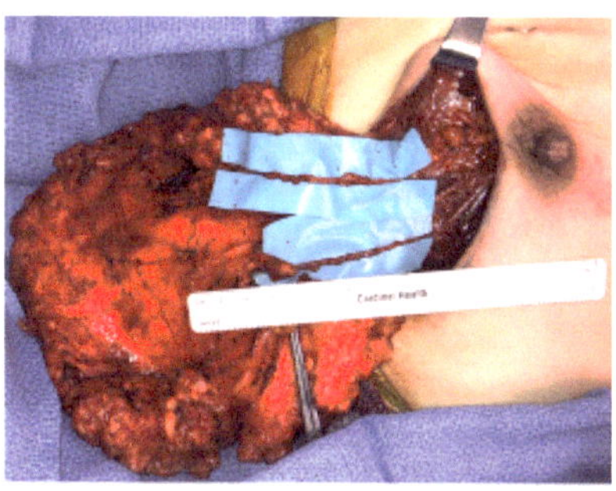

Figure 24.
TRAM flap neurotized to the anterior branch of the third intercostal nerve.

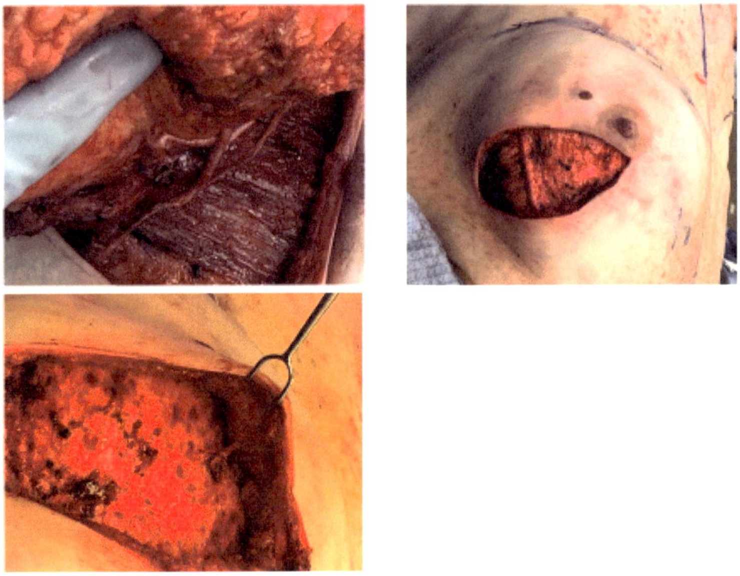

Figure 25.
NAC neurotization to lateral branch of fourth intercostal nerve using nerve graft and tunneled through TRAM flap.

of 37 articles on neurotization of breast reconstruction showed that sensation returns spontaneously but neurotization can lead to earlier return of sensation and increased magnitude [55]. Beside neurotization of the flap, the NAC can be neurotized with the aid of a nerve graft to the lateral branch of the fourth intercostal nerve (**Figure 25**).

9.2 Autologous with implant

Another adjunctive procedure for patients that need flap skin for their breast reconstruction but do not have enough donor tissue volume to reconstruct a larger size breast is the addition of an implant or tissue expander at the time of free tissue transfer [56–60]. This was first reported in 5 patients who had combined TRAM flaps with implants placed by Miller in 1996 [56]. In this study no flap compromise or implant complication

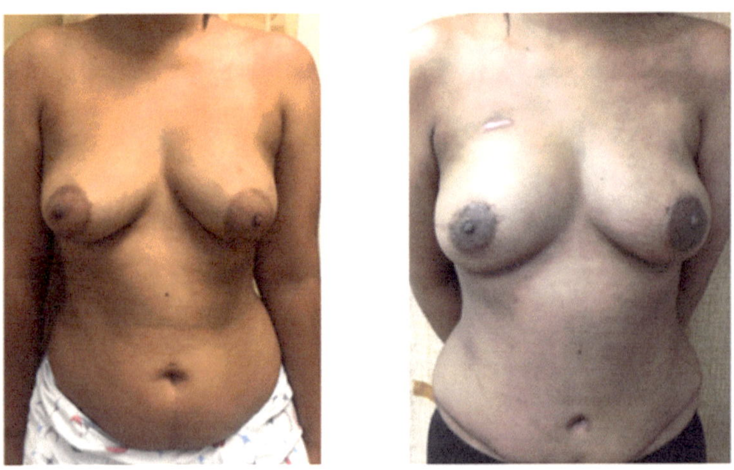

Figure 26.
Bilateral TRAM flap breast reconstruction combined with immediate implant.

was reported. Others have shown that immediate expander/implant placement at the time of the free tissue transfer is associated with higher late (>30 days) implant related complications such as infection, implant rupture, implant malposition, rippling, and capsular contracture [58]. These could be secondary to a longer procedure with unrecognized contamination of the implant and difficulty with forming an appropriate implant pocket [58]. A more recent study by Momeni in 2018 demonstrated that no implant infection, implant malposition, and flap loss occurred in 23 patients that underwent autologous reconstruction with simultaneous prepectoral silicone implant placement [59]. In patients that have undergone neoadjuvant irradiation, the use of TRAM flap combined with an implant significantly lowers the implant loss rate (5 vs. 30%) and reconstruction failures (10 vs. 42%) when compared to expander/implant only reconstructions [60]. Often patients that undergo immediate autologous reconstruction with implant placement have increased esthetic appearance with more breast fullness and less ptosis when compared to their breasts prior to their mastectomies (**Figure 26**).

10. Conclusion

Free autologous tissue transfer from the abdomen is the ideal reconstruction option for the majority of breast cancer patients. The use of autologous tissue can result in a natural appearing breast that is soft, symmetric, and sensate. With improvements in microsurgical techniques, the donor site morbidity and flap complications are minimal allowing for free tissue transfers to be performed in most breast reconstruction patients. Although the abdomen is the preferred donor site, there are other areas that can be utilized for reconstruction. This chapter reviews some of the common free autologous tissue transfers for breast reconstruction along with some adjunctive procedures.

Conflict of interest

The authors have no conflict of interest to disclose.

Notes/thanks/other declarations

The authors would like to thank the division of plastic surgery at Stanford for supporting us in our work.

Author details

Justin Zelones, Suzanne Inchauste and Dung Nguyen*
Stanford University, Palo Alto, California, USA

*Address all correspondence to: nguyendh@stanford.edu

References

[1] Albornoz CR, Back PB, Mehrara BJ, Disa JJ, Pusic AL, McCarthy CM, et al. A paradigm shift in U.S. Breast Reconstruction: Increasing implant rates. Plastic and Reconstructive Surgery. 2013;**131**(1):15-23. DOI: 10.1097/PRS.0b013e3182729cde

[2] Panchal H, Matros E. Current trends in post-mastectomy breast reconstruction. Plastic and Reconstructive Surgery. 2017;**140**(5):7S-13S. DOI: 10.1097/PRS.0000000000003941

[3] Leberfinger AN, Behar BJ, Williams NC, Rakszawski KL, Potochny JD, Mackay DR, et al. Breast implant-associated anaplastic large cell lymphoma: A systematic review. JAMA Surgery. 2017;**152**(12):1161-1168. DOI: 10.1001/jamasurg.2017.4026

[4] Hartrampf CR, Scheflan M, Black PW. Breast reconstruction with a transverse abdominal island flap. Plastic and Reconstructive Surgery. 1982;**69**(2):216-225

[5] Allen RJ, Treece P. Deep inferior epigastric perforator flap for breast reconstruction. Annals of Plastic Surgery. 1994;**32**(1):32-38

[6] Lee BT, Chen C, Nguyen MD, Lin SJ, Tobias AM. A new classification system for muscle and nerve preservation in DIEP flap breast reconstruction. Microsurgery. 2010;**30**(2):85-90. DOI: 10.1002/micr.20717

[7] Lindsey JT. Integrating the DIEP and muscle-sparing (MS-2) free TRAM techniques optimizes surgical outcomes: Presentation of an algorithm for microsurgical breast reconstruction based on perforator anatomy. Plastic and Reconstructive Surgery. 2007;**119**(1):18-27

[8] Chevray PM. Breast reconstruction with superficial inferior epigastric artery flaps: A prospective comparison with TRAM and DIEP flaps. Plastic and Reconstructive Surgery. 2004;**114**(5):1077-1083

[9] Momeni A, Ahdoot MA, Kim RY, Leroux E, Galaia DJ, Lee GK. Should we continue to consider obesity a relative contraindication for autologous microsurgical breast reconstruction? Journal of Plastic, Reconstructive & Aesthetic Surgery. 2012;**65**(4):420-425. DOI: 10.1016/j.bjps.2011.10.005

[10] Moran SL, Salgado CJ, Serletti JM. Free tissue transfer in patients with renal disease. Plastic and Reconstructive Surgery. 2004;**113**(7):2006-2011

[11] Wang TY, Serletti JM, Cuker A, McGrath J, Low DW, Kovach SJ, et al. Free tissue transfer in the hypercoagulable patient: A review of 58 flaps. Plastic and Reconstructive Surgery. 2012;**129**(2):443-453. DOI: 10.1097/PRS.0b013e31823aec4d

[12] Rozen WM, Garcia-Tutor E, Alonso-Burgos A, Corlett RJ, Taylor GI, Ashton MW. The effect of anterior abdominal wall scars on the vascular anatomy of the abdominal wall: A cadaveric and clinical study with clinical implications. Clinical Anatomy. 2009;**22**(7):815-822. DOI: 10.1002/ca.20851

[13] Rozen WM, Ashton MW, Pan WR, Taylor GI. Raising perforator flaps for breast reconstruction: The intramuscular anatomy of the deep inferior epigastric artery. Plastic and Reconstructive Surgery. 2007;**120**(6):1443-1449

[14] Rozen WM, Ashton MW, Stella DL, Phillips TJ, Grinsell D, Taylor GI. The accuracy of computed tomographic angiography for mapping the perforators of the deep inferior epigastric artery. Plastic and Reconstructive Surgery. 2008;**122**(4):1003-1009. DOI: 10.1097/PRS.0b013e3181845994

[15] Tousimis E, Haslinger M. Overview of indications for nipple sparing mastectomy.

Gland Surgery. 2018;**7**(3):288-300. DOI: 10.21037/gs.2017.11.11

[16] Coopey SB, Tang R, Lei L, Freer PE, Kansal K, Colwell AS, et al. Increasing eligibility for nipple-sparing mastectomy. Annals of Surgical Oncology. 2013;**20**(10):3218-3222. DOI: 10.1245/s10434-013-3152-x

[17] Holmstrom H. The free abdominoplasty flap and its use in breast reconstruction. An experimental study and clinical case report. Scandinavian Journal of Plastic and Reconstructive Surgery. 1979;**13**(3):423-427

[18] Mathes SJ, Nahai F. Classification of the vascular anatomy of muscles: Experimental and clinical correlation. Plastic and Reconstructive Surgery. 1981;**67**(2):177-187

[19] Nahabedian MY, Momen B, Galdino G, Manson PN. Breast Reconstruction with the free TRAM or DIEP flap: Patient selection, choice of flap, and outcome. Plastic and Reconstructive Surgery. 2002;**110**(2):466-475

[20] Samargandi OA, Winter J, Corkum JP, Al Youha S, Frank S, Williams J. Comparing the thoracodorsal and internal mammary vessels as recipients for microsurgical autologous breast reconstruction: A systematic review and meta-analysis. Microsurgery. 2017;**37**(8):937-946. DOI: 10.1002/micr.30244

[21] Casey WJ 3rd, Rebecca AM, Smith SS, Craft RO, Buchel EW. The cephalic and external jugular veins: Important alternative recipient vessels in left-sided microvascular breast reconstruction. Microsurgery. 2007;**27**(5):465-469

[22] Fitzgerald O'Connor E, Rozen WM, Chowdhry M, Patel NG, Chow WT, Griffiths M, et al. The microvascular anastomotic coupler for venous anastomoses in free flap breast reconstruction improves outcomes. Gland Surgery. 2016;**5**(2):88-92. DOI: 10.3978/j.issn.2227-684X.2015.05.14

[23] Griffiths M, Chae MP, Rozen WM. Indocyanine green-based fluorescent angiography in breast reconstruction. Gland Surgery. 2016;**5**(2):133-149. DOI: 10.3978/j.issn.2227-684X.2016.02.01

[24] Holm C, Dornseifer U, Sturtz G, Basso G, Schuster T, Ninkovic M. The intrinsic transit time of free microvascular flaps: Clinical and prognostic implications. Microsurgery. 2010;**30**(2):91-96. DOI: 10.1002/micr.20708

[25] Grotting JC. The free abdominoplasty flap for immediate breast reconstruction. Annals of Plastic Surgery. 1991;**27**(4):351-354

[26] Taylor GI, Daniel RK. The anatomy of several free flap donor sites. Plastic and Reconstructive Surgery. 1975;**56**(3):243-253

[27] Nahabedian MY. Breast reconstruction: Free flap techniques. In: Thorne CH, Chung KC, Gosain AK, Gurtner GC, Mehrara BJ, Rubin JP, et al. Grabb and Smith's Plastic Surgery. 7th ed. LWW; 2013. pp. 649-661. Ch. 62

[28] Yousif NJ, Matloub HS, Kolachalam R, Grunert BK, Sanger JR. The transverse gracilis musculocutaneous flap. Annals of Plastic Surgery. 1992;**29**(6):482-490

[29] Arnez ZM, Pogorelec D, Planinsek F, Ahcan U. Breast reconstruction by the free transverse gracilis (TUG) flap. British Journal of Plastic Surgery. 2004;**57**(1):20-26

[30] LoTempio MM, Allen RJ, Blondeel PN. Alternative flaps for breast reconstruction. In: Neligan PC, Geurtner G. Plastic Surgery. 3rd ed. Saunders; 2013. pp. 456-471. Ch. 19

[31] Buntic RF, Horton KM, Brooks D, Althubaiti GA. Transverse upper gracilis flap as an alternative to abdominal tissue breast reconstruction: Technique and modifications. Plastic and Reconstructive Surgery. 2011;**128**(6):607e-613e. DOI: 10.1097/PRS.0b013e318230c2b6

[32] Wechselberger G, Schoeller T. Transverse upper gracilis flap for breast reconstruction. Plastic and Reconstructive Surgery. 2012;**130**(1):182e-183e; author reply183e-184e. DOI: 10.1097/PRS.0b013e318254f606

[33] Haddock NT, Greaney P, Otterburn D, Levine S, Allen RJ. Predicting perforator location on preoperative imaging for the profunda artery perforator flap. Microsurgery. 2012;**32**(7):507-511. DOI: 10.1002/micr.21980

[34] Allen RJ, Haddock NT, Ahn CY, Sadeghi A. Breast reconstruction with the profunda artery perforator flap. Plastic and Reconstructive Surgery. 2012;**129**(1):16e-23e. DOI: 10.1097/PRS.0b013e3182363d9f

[35] Angrigiani C, Grill D, Thorne CH. The adductor flap: A new method for transferring posterior and medial thigh skin. Plastic and Reconstructive Surgery. 2001;**107**(7):1725-1731

[36] Hunter JE, Lardi AM, Dower DR, Farhadi J. Evolution from the TUG to PAP flap for breast reconstruction: Comparison and refinements of technique. Journal of Plastic, Reconstructive & Aesthetic Surgery. 2015;**68**(7):960-965. DOI: 10.1016/j.bjps.2015.03.011

[37] Allen RJ Jr, Lee ZH, Mayo JL, Levine J, Ahn C, Allen RJ Sr. The profunda artery perforator flap experience for breast reconstruction. Plastic and Reconstructive Surgery. 2016;**138**(5):968-975

[38] Fujino T, Harasina T, Aoyagi F. Reconstruction for aplasia of the breast and pectoral region by microvascular transfer of a free flap from the buttock. Plastic and Reconstructive Surgery. 1975;**56**(2):178-181

[39] Allen RJ, Tucker C Jr. Superior gluteal artery perforator free flap for breast reconstruction. Plastic and Reconstructive Surgery. 1995;**95**(7):1207-1212

[40] Hunter C, Moody L, Luan A, Nazerali R, Lee GK. Superior gluteal artery perforator flap: The beauty of the buttock. Annals of Plastic Surgery. 2016;**76**(Suppl 3):S191-S195. DOI: 10.1097/SAP.0000000000000723

[41] Le-Quang C. Secondary microsurgical reconstruction of the breast and free inferior gluteal flap. Annales de Chirurgie Plastique et Esthétique. 1992;**37**(6):723-741

[42] Allen RJ, Levine JL, Granzow JW. The in-the-crease inferior gluteal artery perforator flap for breast reconstruction. Plastic and Reconstructive Surgery. 2006;**118**(2):333-339

[43] Patel NG, Rozen WM, Chow WT, Chowdhry M, Fitzgerald O'Connor E, Sharma H, et al. Stacked and bipedicled abdominal free flaps for breast reconstruction: Considerations for shaping. Gland Surgery. 2016;**5**(2):115-121. DOI: 10.3978/j.issn.2227-684X.2016.02.03

[44] Gorai K, Inoue K, Saegusa N, Shimamoto R, Takeishi M, Okazaki M, et al. Prediction of skin necrosis after mastectomy for breast cancer using indocyanine green angiography imaging. Plastic and Reconstructive Surgery. Global Open. 2017;**5**(4):e1321. DOI: 10.1097/GOX.0000000000001321

[45] Kovach SJ, Georgiade GS. The "banked" TRAM: A method to insure mastectomy skin-flap survival. Annals of Plastic Surgery. 2006;**57**(4):366-369

[46] DellaCroce FJ, Blum CA, Sullivan SK, Stolier A, Trahan C, Wise MW, et al. Nipple-sparing mastectomy and ptosis: Perforator flap breast reconstruction allows full secondary mastopexy with complete nipple areolar repositioning. Plastic and Reconstructive Surgery. 2015;**136**(1):1e-9e. DOI: 10.1097/PRS.0000000000001325

[47] Spear SL, Rottman SJ, Seiboth LA, Hannan CM. Breast reconstruction using a staged nipple-sparing mastectomy following mastopexy or reduction. Plastic and Reconstructive

Surgery. 2012;**129**(3):572-581. DOI: 10.1097/PRS.0b013e318241285c

[48] Al-Mufarrej FM, Woods JE, Jacobson SR. Simultaneous mastopexy in patients undergoing prophylactic nipple-sparing mastectomies and immediate reconstruction. Journal of Plastic, Reconstructive & Aesthetic Surgery. 2013;**66**(6):747-755. DOI: 10.1016/j.bjps.2013.02.007

[49] Rochlin DH, Nguyen DH. Deepithelialized skin reduction preserves skin and nipple perfusion in immediate reconstruction of large and ptotic breasts. Annals of Plastic Surgery. 2018;**81**(1):22-27. DOI: 10.1097/SAP.0000000000001427

[50] Jensen JA, Lin JH, Kapoor N, Giuliano AE. Surgical delay of the nipple-areolar complex: A powerful technique to maximize nipple viability following nipple-sparing mastectomy. Annals of Surgical Oncology. 2012;**19**(10):3171-3176. DOI: 10.1245/s10434-012-2528-7

[51] Bertoni DM, Nguyen D, Rochlin D, Hernandez-Boussard T, Meyer S, Choy N, et al. Protecting nipple perfusion by devascularization and surgical delay in patients at risk for ischemic complications during nipple-sparing mastectomies. Annals of Surgical Oncology. 2016;**23**(8):2665-2672. DOI: 10.1245/s10434-016-5201-8

[52] Dua MM, Bertoni DM, Nguyen D, Meyer S, Gurtner GC, Wapnir IL. Using intraoperative laser angiography to safeguard nipple perfusion in nipple-sparing mastectomies. Gland Surgery. 2015;**4**(6):497-505. DOI: 10.3978/j.issn.2227-684X.2015.04.15

[53] Temple CL, Ross DC, Kim S, Tse R, Bettger-Hahn M, Gan BS, et al. Sensibility following innervated free TRAM flap for breast reconstruction: Part II. Innervation improves patient-rated quality of life. Plastic and Reconstructive Surgery. 2009;**124**(5):1419-1425. DOI: 10.1097/PRS.0b013e3181b98963

[54] Spiegel AJ, Menn ZK, Eldor L, Kaufman Y, Dellon AL. Breast Reinnervation: DIEP neurotization using the third anterior intercostal nerve. Plastic and Reconstructive Surgery. Global Open. 2013;**1**(8):e72. DOI: 10.1097/GOX.0000000000000008

[55] Weissler JM, Koltz PF, Carney MJ, Serletti JM, Wu LC. Sifting through the evidence: A comprehensive review and analysis of neurotization in breast reconstruction. Plastic and Reconstructive Surgery. 2018;**141**(3):550-565. DOI: 10.1097/PRS.0000000000004108

[56] Miller MJ, Rock CS, Robb GL. Aesthetic breast reconstruction using a combination of free transverse rectus abdominis musculocutaneous flaps and breast implants. Annals of Plastic Surgery. 1996;**37**(3):258-264

[57] Serletti JM, Moran SL. The combined use of the TRAM and expanders/implants in breast reconstruction. Annals of Plastic Surgery. 1998;**40**(5):510-514

[58] Roehl KR, Baumann DP, Chevray PM, Chang DW. Evaluation of outcomes in breast reconstructions combining lower abdominal free flaps and permanent implants. Plastic and Reconstructive Surgery. 2010;**126**(2):349-357. DOI: 10.1097/PRS.0b013e3181de1b67

[59] Momeni A, Kanchwala S. Hybrid prepectoral breast reconstruction: A surgical approach that combines the benefits of autologous and implant-based reconstruction. Plastic and Reconstructive Surgery. 2018;**142**(5):1109-1115. DOI: 10.1097/PRS.0000000000004858

[60] Chang DW, Barnea Y, Robb GL. Effects of an autologous flap combined with an implant for breast reconstruction: An evaluation of 1000 consecutive reconstructions of previously irradiated breasts. Plastic and Reconstructive Surgery. 2008;**122**(2):356-362. DOI: 10.1097/PRS.0b013e31817d6303

Chapter 9

Synthetic Mesh in Immediate Breast Reconstruction

Susana Gómez-Modet and Luis Tejedor

Abstract

The use of biological matrices in immediate implant-based breast reconstruction arose with the need to reinforce the lower pole of the breast and to cover the implant to reduce the risk of implant exposure. Synthetic mesh appears to be a lower cost alternative to biological matrices. This literature review aims to assess the usefulness of the use of synthetic meshes in breast reconstruction compared with the traditional techniques and whether outcomes and complications of synthetic meshes and biological matrices are comparable. The positioning of the implants and meshes, either submuscular or subcutaneous, has also been considered.

Keywords: breast cancer, breast reconstruction, synthetic breast meshes, biological breast meshes, complications of breast reconstruction

1. Introduction

Breast cancer is a life-changing diagnosis. Presently, breast conserving therapy can be performed in 70–80% of all breast cancer patients, but in about 20–30% of them mastectomy is indicated as the primary therapeutic management [1–3]. As mastectomy can profoundly affect body image and self-esteem, breast reconstruction should be offered to improve quality of life. Reconstruction may be immediate or delayed, performed with implants or autologous tissue. Immediate reconstruction has several advantages: it provides a psychological benefit, reducing emotional stress and helping to preserve a positive body image [4, 5].

Numerous surgical techniques have been developed, including the use of autologous tissue flaps or silicone implants with or without prior insertion of a tissue expander [1]. Implant-based breast reconstruction (IBBR) accounts for approximately 40–60% of all breast reconstructions in Europe and around 75% in the United States [6]. The American Society of Plastic Surgeons documented a 4% increase in these techniques from 2014 to 2015 and a 35% increase over the last 15 years. A similar trend has also been shown in the United Kingdom, where the rate of IBBR has doubled over the period 1996–2012 [7]. As the number of autologous procedures remains approximately the same, the increased number of immediate procedures can be primarily attributed to an increase in implant/expander reconstructions. This number has substantially increased since skin- and nipple-sparing mastectomies (SSM/NSM) have proven to be oncologically safe procedures.

In IBBR, complete implant coverage has been the mainstay target of surgeons in order to reduce the risk of implant exposure [8]. In the last years, biological and synthetic meshes have emerged as a useful adjunct to breast reconstruction,

IntechOpen

although the decision to add some mesh to an alloplastic reconstruction is controversial. However, there is no high-quality evidence comparing clinical and patient-reported outcomes with mesh-assisted IBBR and traditional IBBR [9]. Finally, the decision for using mesh or not and a particular type of matrix or mesh depends predominately on the surgeons' experience [3, 10].

2. Methods

A literature search has been performed in PubMed, Cochrane, and Embase databases using the keywords "Breast" and "Reconstruction" and "Mesh" and "Synthetic" which rendered 80, 3, and 107 articles, respectively. No date limits were set.

Papers written in English reporting on the complications and/or outcome of IBBR in women aged 18 years or over, either with expander or implants, as a single- or two-stage procedure, either immediate or delayed, both in submuscular and in prepectoral position in which synthetic meshes had been used, were selected for inclusion. Authors screened these articles discarding duplicates, those reporting less than 10 cases, and those unrelated to the subject, leaving a total of 49 papers. The reference list of the retrieved studies was searched manually looking for potentially relevant reports.

3. Synthetic meshes

Usually, the term "matrices" are used for biological materials and the term "meshes" for synthetic materials. There are numerous studies explaining the pros and cons of the matrices, but minimal data are available regarding the synthetic meshes.

Biological meshes or matrices are flexible sheets of tissue that have been stripped of their antigenic cells through a specialised procedure, resulting in decellularisation but leaving the extracellular matrix intact. They provide a scaffold of tissue that the patient's own cells can repopulate and revascularise.

The acellular dermal matrix (ADM), introduced in 1994 [11], is a plate of dermis produced from cadaveric human (Alloderm, Allured, Allomax, Flex HD, Dermacell, Dermamatrix, NeoForm), porcine (Strattice, Permacol, Protexa, XenMartix, XCM), or bovine (SurgiMend) dermis. Other biological meshes come from bovine pericardium (Veritas, Tutopatch, Periguard, Esaflex), porcine peritoneum (Meso Biomatrix), bovine intestine (Surgisis), or fish skin (Kerecis Omega 3 Pectus) [3]. Their utility has been demonstrated in various reconstructive techniques, particularly in burn, abdominal wall repair, and breast reconstruction [11–13].

With the introduction of these meshes, the indications for IBBR became extended, since they provided surgeons with alternative means of obtaining sufficient vascularized soft tissue to cover the implant. Breuing first reported the use of human acellular dermis in IBBR in 2005 [14]. Increased filling volumes of expanders and improved aesthetic outcomes have been reported since then by several authors [4, 15–17]. As new data become available, the use of biological meshes in IBBR will evolve in the following years.

Synthetic meshes are flexible sheets made of plastic-like material that may play a similar role to biological ones in breast reconstruction, becoming an alternative with low cost. The tensile strength of most of these materials is enough to support the physiological demand, although an excessive strength increases inflammation and decreases elasticity. The size of their pores directly impacts on the incorporation of the mesh into the surrounding tissues. Small pores generate a strong inflammatory response that can reduce tissue ingrowth; larger pores allow more ingrowth, preserving elasticity, but promoting more fibrous tissue. Moreover, the mesh can be constructed by knitting or weaving the material. Knitted meshes are generally more porous and flexible than woven meshes that, because of the increased fibre density, are generally stronger and are a poor skeleton for fibrous ingrowth [18].

Besides that, these meshes may be absorbable or non-absorbable. The former are made of polyglycolic acid (Dexon), polyglactin (Vicryl)—both of them are resorbed within a few months—a copolymer of glycolide, lactide and trimethylene carbonate (TIGR Matrix), silk protein (SERI Surgical Scaffold), or a poly-4-hydroxybutyrate polymer (Galatea Scaffold) which is long-term resorbable. Non-absorbable meshes are composed of polypropylene (PP), polyester, (Mersilene), or expanded polytetrafluoroethylene, though just the first material has been used in breast reconstruction (TiLOOP Bra, ULTRAPRO, SERAGYN BR).

3.1 Vicryl

Vicryl mesh is comprised of polyglactin 910 and is a cheap, ready-to-use, and widely available mesh. It causes minimal inflammatory reaction and is non-allergenic and resistant to bacteria biofilm formation. However, because of its rapid resorption, it does not provide a long-lasting tissue reinforcing advantage.

3.2 TiLOOP

This mesh is made of non-resorbable, titanised, lightweight PP with a monofilament structure and was initially invented for hernia repair, showing a good biocompatibility. Production involves introducing titanium in gaseous form so that it reaches all parts of the mesh, forming covalent bonds with the plastic surface. Cellular reactions like proliferation and apoptosis were at the lowest level when using this material compared to not titanium-coated mesh (pure PP), pure lightweight PP mesh, or PP mesh incorporating resorbable polyglactic acid, thus reducing the inflammatory reaction and causing significantly less shrinkage [10]. Clinical studies show that 2 1/2 months after their use, the mesh fibres have been well embedded in the surrounding tissue.

TiLOOP® Bra is intended for extension of the pectoralis major, in the case of subpectoral, implant-based (permanent implant or expander) breast reconstruction. It covers and fixes the caudal pole of the breast implant (**Figure 1**). TiLOOP Bra Pocket is designed to cover a prepectoral implant, providing tissue supporting and preventing displacement.

3.3 SERAGYN BR

The SERAGYN BR mesh is a tightly woven, partially resorbable mesh made of polyglycolic acid-caprolactone and PP. The resorbable part is absorbed within 90–120 days while the non-resorbable part remains in place for additional support. Its biocompatibility is similar to that of the TiLOOP Bra, although surgeons have reported more difficult intraoperative handling due to its firmer characteristics [10].

3.4 ULTRAPRO mesh

ULTRAPRO is manufactured from approximately equal parts of absorbable poliglecaprone-25 monofilament fibre and non-absorbable PP monofilament fibre.

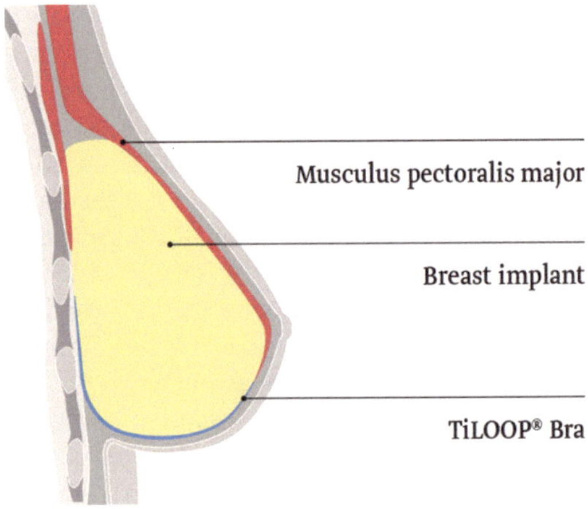

Figure 1.
Tiloop bra.

The absorbable poliglecaprone part of the mesh helps keep the PP structure rigid, thus making intraoperative manipulation and positioning of the mesh easier. The poliglecaprone-25 copolymer is essentially absorbed at 84 days after implantation, remaining only the PP component. Due to the wide pore construction of the mesh, a strong, three-dimensional collagen fibre network is formed [19].

3.5 SERI surgical scaffold

This bioengineered mesh is derived from silk purified to result in ultrapure fibroin (one of the two proteins of the silk). It is a knitted, multifilament, macroporous, and long-term bioresorbable mesh (more than 24 months) intended to resorb slowly, while neovascularization and tissue ingrowth occur. Accordingly, it behaves more like an ADM mesh since it is not just absorbed but accompanied by new tissue generation so that its strength is transferred to the newly ingrown tissue [20].

3.6 TIGR matrix

TIGR Matrix is a long-term resorbable synthetic mesh. The fast-resorbing fibre is a copolymer of lactide, glycolide, and trimethylene carbonate, while the slow-resorbing part is a copolymer of lactide and trimethylene carbonate, completely absorbed after 3 years. Despite its description "matrix" (a term generally used to refer to biological products), the mesh is manufactured synthetically. After implantation, the synthetic fibres degrade at different rates by bulk hydrolysis. It provides additional support in the first 6 months, and complete resorption is achieved after 3 years. In vivo investigations revealed good biocompatibility with the formation of blood vessels and well-structured collagen fibres. The largest series using these meshes is reported by Becker and Lind [21].

3.7 Galatea scaffold

This mesh is made of a poly-4-hydroxybutyrate (P4HB) polymer, which degrades primarily by bulk hydrolysis into a natural metabolite (4HP) that is rapidly metabolised via the Krebs cycle and eliminated as carbon dioxide and water. The mesh is a knitted macroporous scaffold intended to elevate, reinforce, and repair soft tissue. It acts as a lattice for new tissue growth, which is rapidly vascularised and becomes fully integrated with adjacent tissue as the fibres resorb. It retains 50%

of its strength at 16 weeks in vivo and provides a gradual transfer of strength to host tissue over the course of 52 weeks. It is essentially fully resorbed by 18–24 months, allowing the formation of mature strong healthy collagen to support the repair. Its use in breast surgery has recently been described [22].

4. Surgical technique

Primary candidates for mesh reconstruction are patients suited for heterologous breast reconstruction with a small, mid-sized breast and moderate ptosis. Preoperative planning is necessary. Markings must be performed on the day with the patients in an upright position and including the middle and parasternal lines, inframammary folds, and the incision site [23]. There are some possibilities concerning the type of incision technique; in most of the cases, surgeons chose inframammary fold, inverted T, or periareolar.

Prosthetic submuscular IBBR is the most frequent type of reconstruction technique performed nowadays. Placing the implant under the muscular plane traditionally had less major complications than the subcutaneous technique, notwithstanding its burden of pain, limited expansion, implant dislocation, and breast animation. However, adding a mesh to the prepectoral prosthesis allows a complete implant envelope, confers an extra cover, acts as an internal “bra” to relieve pressure on the skin, and defines the implant pocket, preventing lateral displacement. The acceptable complication rate reported in the published studies using this procedure, although with short-term follow-up, has revived this technique [7] (**Figure 2**).

In the submuscular IBBR, after completion of the mastectomy flaps, the inferomedial pectoralis major muscle is elevated for implant placement, serving as a cover towards the maximal thinned out mastectomy flap. Usually, this coverage can often be achieved only for the upper and lower medial quadrant, which can lead to increased implant palpability, with a lack of support and subsequent skin erosion. Although additional coverage can be obtained by mobilising the serratus or the anterior layer of the rectus muscle, this approach involves even more trauma to native tissue and may not be technically possible, particularly in thin patients.

The mesh is fixed to the inferior border of the released pectoral major muscle using running or interrupted resorbable sutures. After placing the implant under the muscle, the mesh is spread over the implant and fixed to the inframammary fold either by single sutures or by wrapping around the implant to gain control of the lower pole [3, 24]. Otherwise, sutures may be given in the opposite order. Mesh

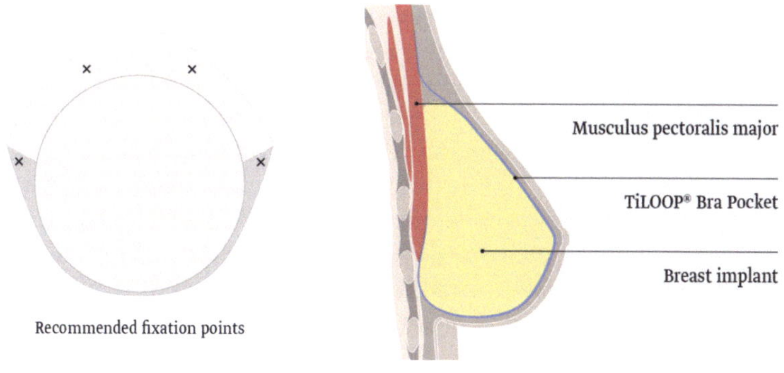

Figure 2.
Recommended implantation procedure in prepectoral reconstruction.

allows to create a more spacious pocket with a natural inframammary fold, bridging the gap between the muscle and chest wall fascia [3, 7] and protecting the pectoralis major from cranial movement.

In the prepectoral IBBR, the mesh or matrix is folded onto itself to create a pocket for the implant or the expander (filled with its final expansion volume and then deflated), and this pocket is sutured to the pectoral major fascia with at least three stitches, apical, medial, and lateral [25]. Advantages of this approach include less tissue dissection, less postoperative pain, better filling of the medial breast, avoidance of lateral fallout, and absence of hyperanimation deformity. This technique is frequently used in combination with new technologies such as autologous fat grafting and perfusion analysis of the skin flaps.

5. Complications

Mesh use in breast reconstruction is associated with many complications. Infection, seroma, hematoma, capsular contracture, skin flap necrosis, explantation or implant loss are the most commonly reported. Of course, some characteristics of patients are associated with increased complication rates, with or without use of a mesh. These include age (older than 65 years), large breasts (more than 600 g), obesity (BMI greater than 30), smoking, diabetes, hypertension, long drain removal time, previous radiotherapy to the ipsilateral breast, and receipt of neoadjuvant chemotherapy [1, 2].

Infection is one of the most common complications seen in both biological and synthetic mesh use, which often leads to tissue necrosis and may result in explantation, revision, or even complete loss of implant [1, 26]. Ellis et al. reported rates of infection shifting between 0.2 and 35.8%, the higher numbers seen after ADM use [1, 2]. A high-throughput assay comparing synthetic meshes (Prolene and Vicryl) and biological matrices (Alloderm and Flex HD) as substrates for bacterial adhesion concluded that *Staphylococcus aureus* adhered more readily to ADMs than to meshes, therefore showing a greater potential propensity for biofilm development [27].

Seroma and haematoma are commonly occurring complications and can both lead to an increased risk of infection and tissue necrosis, particularly when large enough to require drain insertion. Haematoma formation is thought to occur in the immediate postoperative period as a result of trauma during surgery—although the use of electrocautery has significantly reduced its incidence—or as a late complication due to small tears in the capsule formed around the implant, often after physical trauma [1]. There seems to be different seroma formation rates between the two types of meshes. Matrices have smooth surfaces, allowing increased fluctuation between the matrix and the subcutaneous tissue and resulting in the development of seromas. Meshes have rougher surfaces and thus a potentially faster interaction with the subcutaneous tissue, lesser fluctuation, and a consequent decrease in seroma formation [10]. Rates are between 0 and 5.7% for meshes and between 1.5 and 24.3 for ADM [1].

Capsular contracture is described as the formation of a fibrous capsule around the implant that thickens progressively and may contract, compressing the implant and resulting in a hard breast with deformed contouring of the surrounding skin. This may also cause severe pain due to nerve entrapment or muscle mobility interference. Although the aetiology is unclear, some believe that it is initiated by blood products like haematomas, while others consider infection and chronic inflammation to be most likely the cause, either by bacteria colonisation from within the ductal breast tissue or from the skin [1, 28]. Studies have reported significantly lower rates of capsular contracture with the use of ADM than without it, but the length of the follow-up is short [20]. Although no high-quality study has directly compared the incidence of capsular contracture between synthetic and biological matrices IBBR, rates are similar for both types (1.3–8.6% for meshes and 0.4–8.1% for matrices) [1, 3, 28, 29]. Dieterich et al. [30] reported a histological analysis with mild inflammation using TiLOOP, suggesting a low risk of capsular contracture.

Loss of vascular supply to the overlying mastectomy skin flap is the reason of skin necrosis after ischaemic changes. This is a multifactorial event: patient comorbidities, thin mastectomy skin flaps, or over expansion may contribute [1]. Regarding the surgical technique, rates of skin necrosis up to 30% have been associated with the use of inverted T-incision, especially at the T-junction [24].

Rates of 1.8–4.3% for meshes and 1.4–24.3% for matrices have been published [1].

All of the above complications, if severe enough, may lead to implant explantation, often resulting in complete implant loss. Most of the studies showed comparable rates of implantation loss using matrices or synthetic meshes (between 0 and 8.7%), although some reports explantation rates as high as 33.3% for ADM [1, 29].

6. Discussion

Reconstructive breast techniques with expander or implant without biologic or synthetic meshes can have disadvantages. In the short run, they may present with a thin or insufficient coverage of the implant, a risky stress of the inferior pole along with a decreased skin perfusion with a too early or too extensive expansion, and a herniation and sequential skin erosion towards the lateral border of the pectoralis major muscle or the inferior pole. In the medium and long term, a high-riding implant due to muscle stiffness, a restricted expansion of the inferior pole, or a loss of definition of the inframammary fold may appear. By using these meshes to support and cover these weak points, these disadvantages can be diminished or even resolved [30].

Benefits of their use include improved coverage over the device, lengthening and support of the pectoralis muscle, support for the lower pole, more rapid expansion, improved definition of the breast boundaries and folds, and possible modification of capsule formation. Disadvantages include added risk of infection, seroma formation, risk of flap necrosis and implant exposure, added surgical time, and increased cost [31, 32]. These complications may be higher than traditional implant reconstruction, and there is no yet evidence on long-term outcomes of these mesh procedures, including the need for further surgery over time [33].

Although the choice of using a mesh or a matrix is controversial and depends basically on individual surgeon preference, there are indications where matrices may be advisable, such as in revisional breast surgery or after irradiation, since reported data suggest a better blood flow to the irradiated skin and, for some author, a decreased rate of capsular contracture compared with meshes [24]. Published guidelines, though largely based on poor-quality evidence and expert opinion, offer sensible advice regarding current best practice. The American Society of Plastic Surgeons recommends using mesh on a per patient basis. The United Kingdom professional associations (Association of Breast Surgery and the British Association of Plastic, Reconstructive, and Aesthetic Surgeons) advocate careful patient selection and employing mesh-assisted IBBR with caution in high-risk groups (current smokers, previous breast radiotherapy, high BMI) [21, 34]. A joint consensus guide on prepectoral IBBR from European and US surgeons has been recently published [35]. After a systematic review, Cabalag et al. offer a summary of recommendations for ADM use [36].

Regarding outcomes when using these materials, a recent systematic review noted a higher rate of infection with mesh-assisted IBBR than traditional IBBR, but the quality of evidence is low [37]. Improved cosmetic results have been advocated for the use of matrices, although the outcomes of the reported studies are of limited value [20, 29]. Sigalove et al. found less than 5% of aesthetic complications (capsular contracture, implant malposition, and rippling) after prepectoral reconstruction with ADM. Their complication rate was 9.1%: 4.5% infections, 2.0% seromas, and 2.5% necrosis [38]. Obtaining data from 14,249 patients, Pannucci et al. reported a significant increased risk of 0.7% (1.85 vs. 2.58%) expander/implant loss when ADM was used [39].

Salibian et al. showed 85.2% of patients as having very good or good results with prepectoral expander/implant without any additional material (together with infection in 2.4%, necrosis in 6.8%, capsular contracture Baker grade III or IV in 7.6%, and rippling in 3.6% of the patients) [40].

In a small pilot randomised controlled trial comparing biological and synthetic meshes, Gschwantler-Kaulich et al. [24] found no statistically significant differences in cosmetic outcome and overall complications between the groups, but patients in the ADM group experienced substantially higher rates of implant loss than those undergoing IBBR with synthetic mesh (although the first group was more exposed to radiotherapy). Nevertheless, this study is insufficiently designed to look at the target difference between the treatment groups and is of very low-quality evidence.

A recent cohort study reported no differences in satisfaction and quality of life between the use of matrix (Surgisis) or mesh (TIGR) in IBBR [41]. Reitsemer et al. reported low complication rates after 200 prepectoral reconstructions with the use of ADM or TIGR mesh, but with no comparison between both [42]. A systematic review comparing subcutaneous IBBR using ADM or meshes (without any information about the types of meshes) concluded that short-term complication rates are low and similar but refers that statistical analysis was not possible given differing study designs, confounding variables, and lack of comparative data in each study [43].

In a retrospective cohort study comparing the benefits of mesh (TiLOOP) versus non-mesh reconstructions, there was no statistical significance either in complications or in patient-reported outcomes [3]. In a large retrospective multicenter study of 231 procedures using synthetic mesh (TiLOOP Bra), Dieterich revealed major complications (those needing additional surgery) occurring in 13.4%, minor complications (requiring just conservative measures) in 15.6%, and implant loss in 8.7% of patients. The overall infection rate was 6.1% of which only 1.7% needed revision, and the seroma rate was 4.8%. In this chapter, risk factors for postoperative complications included a bilateral procedure or a previous skin expansion. The authors concluded that these were acceptable complication rates, that the mesh should only be used in primary cases, and that, when adhering to the proposed indications, it was a safe and convenient option in implant-based breast reconstruction [26].

Low complication rates (6.6%, including implant loss of 1.3%) and good aesthetic results have also been reported by Tessler et al. with the use of Vicryl meshes, which add to their economic advantage over matrices, but again with insufficient power to obtain clear-cut conclusions [44].

Hallberg et al. noticed complications in 23% of the patients with IBBR using TIGR Matrix, including two implant losses. Reported risk factors were age over 51 years, BMI over 24.5 kg/m2, large resection weight, and a Wise pattern excision of the skin [45]. A similar rate of complications with the same material was stated by Pompei et al., with 11.6% of the patients requiring revisional surgery but with removal of the mesh only in 3.3% of them. These authors found that this mesh caused low seroma (3.6%) and infection rates (1.6%) when compared with other nonreabsorbable or semiresorbable synthetic meshes, but also this study has a low quality of evidence [46]. A recent abstract reports on 34 patients reconstructed with TIGR Matrix encountered 9% cases with infections, 9% with necrosis, 5.9% with seromas, and 3% with reoperations [47]. Schrenk et al. found just one case of seroma and another of skin necrosis, needing reoperation, after 37 IBBR with the same mesh [48]. Irwin et al. had 11 implant losses out of 94 cases with the same material [49].

In a prospective study with 187 patients treated with prepectoral expander and TiLOOP Bra mesh and with a mean follow-up of 36.5 months, Casella et al. found complications requiring a second operation in 6.7% of the cases, with implant loss in half of them. Capsular contracture, implant malposition, and, above all, rippling appeared in 16.4%. Patients scored a high level of satisfaction [50].

In a study comparing reconstruction with a prepectoral titanium mesh wrap to subpectoral titanium sling, there was only one implant failure in the prepectoral cohort. There were no significant differences between the two groups with any complication, including infection, implant loss, skin necrosis, hematoma, or reoperation at 1-year follow-up [51]. Two-year follow-up demonstrated no capsular contracture in the prepectoral cohort and 12% in the partial subpectoral cohort [52]. Other paper by Casella et al. on 250 cases of prepectoral implant immediate reconstruction and TiLOOP recounts complications in 2.4% of the cases, but aesthetic complications are brought to reoperations in 19.5% of the breasts [53].

A reported side effect of titanium-coated permanent mesh in IBBR is the formation of granulomas in the inframammary fold, probably in the area where the mesh had been folded or fixed, mimicking a local recurrence [54]. Other papers state good cosmetic results and/or a low rate of complications with the use of this mesh [3, 55, 56].

A retrospective analysis of 320 cases comparing TiLOOP Bra mesh with SERAGYN mesh reported no differences in complication rates (and no differences in performance when compared to ADM) [58, 59]. A similar report about 131 patients with SERAGYN showed a rate of complication comparable to the use of other meshes or matrices (seroma in 25.7%, reconstructive failure in 11.5%, wound healing issues in 13.5%, wound infections in 10.8%), without severe complications in 83.8% of operations [60]. Other retrospective study with 102 patients and 174 IBBR using ULTRAPRO, which included 45.1% patients with previous radiotherapy and pre-existing scars, recorded complications in 18.3%, (6.9% minor and 11.4% major, requiring revision) [19]. A similar report with 70 cases of reconstructed breast using SURGIMESH found no statistical significances in outcomes compared with standard IBBR without meshes [61]. Another paper about the use of polyester mesh (Mersilene) in 73 patients reported an explantation rate of 4.1%, although the surgical technique included an abdominal advancement flap [62]. One abstract reported similar results with polyester mesh, titanium mesh, and ADM in 104 cases, with excellent results in 67.3% of them [63].

The best report till the date is a prospective, multicentre cohort study in the United Kingdom, where 2108 patients were recruited to establish the short-term safety of immediate IBBR performed with and without mesh, either biological or synthetic, in prepectoral or submuscular pockets. After 3 months of surgery, 9% of the patients suffered implant loss, 18% required readmission, 18% needed a second surgery because of the complications, and 25% had treatment for an infection, with no differences regarding mesh use or type [2]. This analysis also identified an association between infection and previous radiotherapy. Ages, neoadjuvant chemotherapy, bilateral surgery, indication for surgery, nipple-sparing procedure,

Ref. No	Surgical technique	Mesh type	Breasts no.	Infection	Explantation	Necrosis	Seroma/ hematoma	Contracture grade III–IV	Reoperation	Total	Aesthetic Ex+G	RT
[2]	All	ADM	1133	22.0	8.0				17.0			7.0
		TiLOOP	243	26.0	10.0				20.0			
[3]	All	TiLOOP	48	6.0		4.1	2/0	4.1	6.0	21.1	NS	
		None	42	14.2		14.2	6/4.1	16.6	4.1	28.6		
[8]	Submuscular	TIGR	54	1.7		5.0	3.3/6.7	1.7	11.6	23.3		10.2
[9]		TiLOOP	79		6.0					18.0		
		Strattice	35		6.0					22.0		
[19]	Submuscular	ULTRAPRO	174	4.5		4.0	5.1/1.2	1.2	6.3	18.3		41.5
[21]	Revisional	TIGR	112	3.6		1.8	1.8		15.2	20.5		14.5
[22]		P4HB	110	8.0	6.0							28.0
		ADM	198	15.0	8.0							37.0
[24]		Protexa	25*	12.0	30.4		12.0			39.1	79.0	16.0
		TiLOOP	23*	4.3	7.7		4.3/8.6			24.0	87.5	0.0
[26]	Submuscular	TiLOOP	231	6.1	8.7	4.3	4.8/9.5	2.2		29.0		2.1
[41]		Surgisis	116		15.1			5.5		35.8	NS	
		TIGR	65		4.9			4.9		29.3		
[42]	Prepectoral	ADM and TIGR	200		3.5		0.0/4.0	0.0			90.0	13.0
[44]	Submuscular	Vicryl	76	1.3	1.3	2.6	0.0/0.0	1.3	3.9	6.6		18.4
[45]	Submuscular	TIGR	65	1.5	3.1	1.5	3.1/1.5		1.5	23.2		
[46]	Submuscular	TIGR	54	1.7		5.0	3.3/6.7	1.7	11.6			10.2
[47]	All	TIGR	40	7.5		7.5	5.0/0.0					22.5
[48]	Submuscular expander	TiLOOP	237	2.5		1.3	1.2/0.0	3.8	6.7		BREAST-Q 1	26.5

DOI: http://dx.doi.org/10.5772/intechopen.90884

Ref. No	Surgical technique	Mesh type	Breasts no.	Infection	Explantation	Necrosis	Seroma/ hematoma	Contracture grade III–IV	Reoperation	Total	Aesthetic Ex+G	RT
[49]	Submuscular	TiLOOP	34	5.8	0.0	0.0	0.0/0.0					
	Prepectoral		39	0.0	2.5	2.5	0.0/2.5					
[51]	Prepectoral	TiLOOP	250	0.8	1.2	0.8	0.0/0.4	4.0	2.4		BREAST-Q 2	7.2
[53]		TiLOOP	87*	10.3			9.2/17.2					
[57]	Submuscular	TiLOOP	269*			0.7		0.3			BREAST-Q 3	9.7
[60]	All	SERAGYN	148	14.2		8.1	25.7/14.2	1.4	22.9			17.6
[19]	Submuscular	ULTRAPRO	174	4.5		4.0	5.1/1.2	1.2	11.4			45.1
[61]	Submuscular	SURGIMESH	70	10.0	7.1	10.0	8.5/1.4	7.1				12.7
		None	136	5.88	10.0	10.0	7.3/0.0					
[62]	Submuscular	Mersilene	73*	1.4	4.1			13.6	19.2		77.5	

Aesthetic Ex+G: aesthetic results excellent and goods.
RT: % of cases with pre- and postoperative radiotherapy.
NS: not significant.
**Number of patients (number of cases not reported).*
BREAST-Q 1: overall satisfaction with outcome 74.0, satisfaction with breasts 72.2, psychosocial wellness 77.5, and sexual well-being 61.6.
BREAST-Q 2: overall satisfaction with outcome 73.8, satisfaction with breasts 72.5, psychosocial wellness 77.7, and sexual well-being 57.9.
BREAST-Q 3: overall satisfaction with outcome 74.8, satisfaction with breasts 60.2, psychosocial wellness 71.3, and sexual well-being 56.4.

Table 1.
Number of complications is given in percentage.

fixed-volume implant, and type of reconstruction were not significant risk factors. A summary of all these data is shown in **Table 1**. A number of studies are currently underway in Europe [64].

It is well known that radiotherapy has a significantly detrimental effect on most breast reconstruction outcomes, whether given pre- or postoperatively (but without differences in complication rates between both) [65], since it impedes neovascularisation and mesh incorporation into the host [1]. Most published studies identify radiotherapy as adversely affecting the cosmetic outcome by precipitating the inflammatory reaction of the implant to the surrounding tissues. Becker described frequent complications in patients that received radiotherapy and were reconstructed with TIGR mesh [21]. Similar results were reported by Dieterich et al. using TiLOOP mesh [26] and by others using ADM [1, 4, 66–68]. On the other hand, some protective effects of matrices against radiotherapy, compared with those patients without them, have been reported, since biological meshes appear to limit the elastosis and chronic inflammation seen in irradiated IBBR [69, 70].

To sum up, the literature on this subject is difficult to interpret because there is neither high-quality evidence comparing outcomes of mesh-assisted IBBR with traditional IBBR or comparing matrices with meshes. Most studies in this area are small, single-centre, retrospective cohort studies and case series with methodological limitations: different surgical techniques, with different meshes and matrices, differing in sizes and positions, with very disparate ways of reporting complications (in fact, it is often unclear what complications have been included and how they have been diagnosed and how and when capsular contracture and aesthetic outcome have been evaluated), thus carrying a low level of evidence [37]. Randomised clinical trials with sufficient periods of follow-up should be carried out to determine whether the cost of these products is justified in terms of the benefits provided [71].

7. Conclusions

Although it is still unclear whether mesh procedures are a safe alternative to traditional IBBR regarding patient-reported outcomes, matrices and meshes have proven to wear valuable advantages. Moreover, there is not even a consensus on which of the two types produces the best outcomes, although there is a trend to consider that meshes bring comparable aesthetic outcomes to matrices, with lower costs and complication rates. Regarding the uncertainty about the best position for the implant, either submuscular or subcutaneous, the prepectoral position is gaining ground quickly among surgeons and patients.

Most of the literature have focused on the complication and safety profiles of these meshes, but, given that the purpose of breast reconstruction is to improve body image and psychosocial function, it is equally important that cosmesis and patient satisfaction are also included when evaluating the results of these techniques.

Conflict of interest

The authors declare no conflict of interest.

Author details

Susana Gómez-Modet and Luis Tejedor*
Punta Europa Hospital, Algeciras, Spain

*Address all correspondence to: tejedor@comcadiz.es

References

[1] Ellis HL, Asaolu O, Nebo V, et al. Biological and synthetic mesh use in breast reconstructive surgery: A literature review. World Journal of Surgical Oncology. 2016;**14**:121. DOI: 10.1186/s12957-016-0874-9

[2] Potter S, Conroy EJ, Cutress RI, et al. Short-term safety outcomes of mastectomy and immediate implant-based breast reconstruction with and without mesh (iBRA): A multicentre, prospective cohort study. The Lancet Oncology. 2019;**20**:254-266

[3] Dieterich M, Angres J, Stachs A, et al. Patient-report satisfaction and health-related quality of life in tiloop bra- assisted or implant-based breast reconstruction alone. Aesthetic Plastic Surgery. 2015;**39**:523-533

[4] Spear SL, Parikh PM, Reisin E, et al. Acellular dermis-assisted breast reconstruction. Aesthetic Plastic Surgery. 2008;**32**:418-425

[5] Nava M. Breast reconstruction with form-stable implants. In: Surgery of the Breast, Principles and Art. 3rd ed. Vol. 36. 2011. pp. 429-437

[6] Paepke S, Ohlinger R, Klein E, et al. Prepectoral implant placement in plastic-reconstructive breast surgery- a contribution to the discussion. Senology. 2018;**15**:115-119

[7] Tasoulis MK, Iqbal FM, Cawthorn S, et al. Subcutaneous implant breast reconstruction: Time to reconsider? European Journal of Surgical Oncology. 2017;**43**:1636-1646

[8] Pompei S, Evangelidou D, Arelli F, et al. The use of TIGR matrix in breast aesthetic and reconstructive surgery. Is a resorbable synthetic mesh a viable alternative to acellular dermal matrices? Clinics in Plastic Surgery. 2018;**45**:65-73

[9] McKenna A, Hamilton-Burke W, Bathia S, et al. A comparative study of titanium-coated propylene mesh with acellular dermal matrix in implant based breast reconstruction. European Journal of Surgical Oncology. 2017;**43**:S47. DOI: 10.1016/j.ejso.2017.01.180

[10] Dieterich M, Faridi A. Biological matrices and synthetic meshes used in implant-based breast reconstruction- a review of products available in Germany. Geburtshilfe und Frauenheilkunde. 2013;**73**:1100-1106

[11] Wainwright DJ. Use of an acellular allograft dermal matrix (AlloDerm) in the management of full-thickness burns. Burns. 1995;**21**(4):243-248

[12] Butler CE, Langstein HN, Kronowitz SJ. Pelvic, abdominal, and chest wall reconstruction with AlloDerm in patients at increased risk for mesh-related complications. Plastic and Reconstructive Surgery. 2005;**116**(5):263-275

[13] Chaplin JM, Costantino PD, Wolpoe ME, et al. Use of an acellular dermal allograft for dural replacement: An experimental study. Neurosurgery. 1999;**45**(2):320-327

[14] Breuing KH, Warren SM. Immediate bilateral breast reconstruction with implants and inferolateral AlloDerm slings. Annals of Plastic Surgery. 2005;**55**(3):232-239

[15] Salzberg CA. Nonexpansive immediate breast reconstruction using human acellular tissue matrix graft (AlloDerm). Annals of Plastic Surgery. 2006;**57**(1):1-5

[16] Bindingnavele V, Gaon M, Ota KS, et al. Use of acellular cadaveric dermis and tissue expansion in postmastectomy breast reconstruction. Journal of Plastic, Reconstructive & Aesthetic Surgery. 2007;**60**(11):1214-1218

[17] Preminger BA, McCarthy CM, Hu QY, et al. The influence of AlloDerm on expander dynamics and complications in the setting of immediate tissue expander/implant reconstruction: A matched-cohort study. Annals of Plastic Surgery. 2008;**60**(5):510-513

[18] Fitzgerald JF, Kumar AS. Biologic versus synthetic mesh reinforcement: What are the pros and cons? Clinics in Colon and Rectal Surgery. 2014;**27**(4):140-148. DOI: 10.1055/s-0034-1394155

[19] Pukancsik D, Kelemen P, Gulyás G, et al. Clinical experiences with the use of ULTRAPRO mesh in single-stage direct-to-implant immediate postmastectomy breast reconstruction in 102 patients: A retrospective cohort study. European Journal of Surgical Oncology. 2017;**47**:1244-1251

[20] Cook LJ, Kovacs T. Novel devices for implant-based breast reconstruction: Is the use of meshes to support the lower pole justified in terms of benefits? A review of the evidence. Ecancermedicalscience. 2018;**10**(12):796. DOI: 10.3332/ecancer.2018.796

[21] Becker H, Lind JG. The use of synthetic mesh in reconstructive, revision, and cosmetic breast surgery. Aesthetic Plastic Surgery. 2013;**37**:914-921

[22] Levy AS, Bernstein JL, Otter-burn DM. Biosynthetic mesh compares favorably to ADM in tissue expander-based breast reconstruction. Plastic and Reconstructive Surgery. Global Open. 2017;**5**(48):86-87. DOI: 10.1097/01.GOX.0000516637.00470.c0

[23] de Vita R, Buccheri EM, Villanucci A, et al. Breast reconstruction actualized in nipple-sparing mastectomy and direct-to-implant, prepectoral polyurethane positioning: Early experience and preliminary results. Clinical Breast Cancer. 2019;**19**(2):e358-e363

[24] Gschwantler-Kaulich D, Schrenk P, Bjelic-Radisic V, et al. Mesh versus acellular dermal matrix in immediate implant-based breast reconstruction-a prospective randomized trial. European Journal of Surgical Oncology. 2016;**42**:665-671

[25] Marcasciano M, Kaliulyte J, Gen Tilucci M, et al. Skin-reduction breast reconstructions with prepectoral implant covered by a combined dermal flap and titanium-coated polypropylene mesh. Journal of Plastic, Reconstructive & Aesthetic Surgery. 2018;**71**(8):1123-1128. DOI: 10.1016/j.bjps.2018.05.005

[26] Dieterich M, Paepke S, Zwiefel K, et al. Implant-based breast reconstruction using a titanium-coated polypropylene mesh (TiLOOP bra): a multicenter study of 231 cases. Plastic and Reconstructive Surgery. 2013;**132**:8e-19e

[27] Nyame TT, Lemon KP, Kolter R, et al. High-throughput assay for bacterial adhesion on acellular dermal matrices and synthetic surgical materials. Plastic and Reconstructive Surgery. 2011;**128**:1061-1068

[28] Bengtson B. Discussion: Use of dermal matrix to prevent capsular contracture in aesthetic breast surgery. Plastic and Reconstructive Surgery. 2012;**130**:1374-1375

[29] Wagner RD, Braun TL, Zhu H, et al. A systematic review of complications in prepectoral breast reconstruction. Journal of Plastic, Reconstructive & Aesthetic Surgery. 2019;**72**:1051-1059

[30] Dieterich M, Dieterich H, Timme S, et al. Using a titanium-coated polypropylene mesh (TiLOOP (R)) bra for implant-based breast reconstruction: Case report and histological analysis.

Archives of Gynecology and Obstetrics. 2012;**286**:273-276

[31] Kim JYS, Davila AA, Persing S, et al. A meta-analysis of human acellular dermis and submuscular tissue expander breast reconstruction. Plastic and Reconstructive Surgery. 2012;**129**(1):28-41. DOI: 10.1097/PRS.0b013e3182361fd6

[32] Brown M, Namnoum JD. Indications and controversies for implant-only based breast reconstruction. Clinics in Plastic Surgery. 2018;**45**:47-54

[33] Potter S, MacKenzie M, Blazeby JN. Does the addition of mesh improve outcomes in implant based breast reconstruction after mastectomy for breast cancer? BMJ. 2018;**362**:k2607. DOI: 10.1136/bmj.k2607

[34] Martin L, O'Donoghuc JM, Horgan K, et al. Acellular dermal matrix (ADM) assisted breast reconstruction procedures: Joint guidelines from the Association of Breast Surgery and the British Association of Plastic, Reconstructive and Aesthetic Surgeons. European Journal of Surgical Oncology. 2013;**39**(5):425-429. DOI: 10.1016/j.ejso.2012.12.012

[35] Vidya R, Berna G, Sbitany H, et al. Prepectoral implant-based breast reconstruction: A joint consensus guide from UK, European and USA breast and plastic reconstructive surgeons. ecancer. 2019;**13**:927. DOI: 10.3332/ecancer.2019.927

[36] Cabalag MS, Rostek M, Miller GS, et al. Alloplastic adjuncts in breast reconstruction. Gland Surgery. 2016;**5**(2):158-173. DOI: 10.3978/j.issn.2227-684X.2015.06.02

[37] Hallberg H, Rafnsdottir S, Selvaggi G, et al. Benefits and risks with acellular dermal matrix (ADM) and mesh support in immediate breast reconstruction: a systematic review and meta-analysis. Journal of Plastic Surgery and Hand Surgery. 2018;**52**:130-147. DOI: 10.1080/2000656X.2017.1419141. 29320921

[38] Sigalove S, Maxwell GP, Sigalove NM, et al. Prepectoral implant-based breast reconstruction: Rationale, indications, and preliminary results. Plastic and Reconstructive Surgery. 2017;**139**:287-294

[39] Pannucci CJ, Antony AK, Wilkins EG. The impact of acellular dermal matrix on tissue expander/implant loss in breast reconstruction: An analysis of the tracking outcomes and operations in plastic surgery database. Plastic and Reconstructive Surgery. 2013;**132**(1):1-10. DOI: 10.1097/PRS.0b013e318290f917

[40] Salibian AH, Harness JK, Mowlds DS. Staged suprapectoral expander/implant reconstruction without acellular dermal matrix following nipple-sparing mastectomy. Plastic and Reconstructive Surgery. 2017;**139**(1):30-39. DOI: 10.1097/PRS.0000000000002845

[41] Hallberg H, Flander a KL, et al. A biological or a synthetic mesh in immediate breast reconstruction? A cohort study of long-term health related quality of life (HrQoL). European Journal of Surgical Oncology. 2019;**45**(10):1812-1816. DOI: 10.1016/j.ejso.2019.03.013

[42] Reitsamer R, Peintinger F, Klaassen-Federspiel F, et al. Prepectoral direct-to-implant breast reconstruction with complete ADM or synthetic mesh coverage. 36-months follow-up in 200 reconstructed breasts. Breast. 2019;**48**:32-37. DOI: 10.1016/j.breast.2019.08.002

[43] Salibian AH, Frey JD, Choi M, et al. Subcutaneous implant-based breast reconstruction with acellular dermal matrix/mesh: A systematic review.

Plastic and Reconstructive Surgery Global Open. 2016;**23**(4):11, e1139. DOI: 10.1097/GOX.0000000000001139

[44] Tessler O, Reish RG, Maman DY, et al. Beyond biologics: Absorbable mesh as a low-cost, low-complication sling for implant-based breast reconstruction. Plastic and Reconstructive Surgery. 2014;**133**(2):90e-99e. DOI: 10.1097/01.prs.0000437253.55457.6339

[45] Hallberg H, Lewin R, Elander A, et al. TIGR® matrix surgical mesh—A two-year follow-up study and complication analysis in 65 immediate breast reconstructions. Journal of Plastic Surgery and Hand Surgery. 2018;**52**(4):253-258. DOI: 10.1080/2000656X.2018.1478841

[46] Pompei S, Evangelidou D, Arrelli F, et al. The use of TIGR matrix in breast aesthetic and reconstructive surgery. Is a reabsorbable synthetic mesh a viable alternative to acellular dermal matrices? Clinics in Plastic Surgery. 2018;**45**:65-73. DOI: 10.1016/j.cps.2017.08.005

[47] Cuffolo G, Holford N, Contractor K, et al. TIGR matrix synthetic long-term reabsorbable mesh for prepectoral and subpectoral implant based breast reconstruction: Outcomes of two years practice. European Journal of Surgical Oncology. 2019;**45**(5):915. DOI: 10.1016/j.ejso.2019.01.138

[48] Schrenk P. Immediate implant-based breast reconstruction using the TIGR® matrix mesh. Breast Cancer Management. 2016;**5**(2):53-59

[49] Irwin G, Darragh L, Mallon P, et al. TIGR matrix mesh in breast reconstruction. A single unit experience. European Journal of Surgical Oncology. 2017;**43**(5):S24. DOI: 10.1016/j.ejso.2017.01.099

[50] Casella D, Di Taranto G, Marcasciano M, et al. Subcutaneous expanders and synthetic mesh for breast reconstruction: Long-term and patient-reported BREAST-Q outcomes of a single-center prospective study. Journal of Plastic, Reconstructive & Aesthetic Surgery. 2019;**72**(5):805-812. DOI: 10.1016/j.bjps.2018.12.018

[51] Casella D, Bernini M, Bencini L, et al. TiLoop® bra mesh used for immediate breast reconstruction: Comparison of retropectoral and subcutaneous implant placement in a prospective single-institution series. European Journal of Plastic Surgery. 2014;**37**(11):599-604

[52] Bernini M, Calabrese C, Cecconi L, et al. Subcutaneous direct-to-implant breast reconstruction: Surgical, functional, and aesthetic results after long-term follow-up. Plastic and Reconstructive Surgery. Global Open;**3**(12):-e574

[53] Casella D, Di Taranto G, Marcasciano M, et al. Evaluation of prepectoral implant placement and complete coverage with TiLoop bra mesh for breast reconstruction: A prospective study on long-term and patient-reported BREAST-Q outcomes. Plastic and Reconstructive Surgery. 2019;**143**(1):1e-9e. DOI: 10.1097/PRS.0000000000005078

[54] Riggio E, Chifu C, Martelli G, et al. Can titanium mesh influence local recurrence management after implant-based breast reconstruction? Springerplus. 2015;**4**(4):482. DOI: 10.1186/s40064-015-1273-3

[55] Klein E, Kiechle M, Paepke S. Analysis of immediate breast reconstruction with the use of titanized polypropylene mesh (TiLOOP® bra). European Journal of Surgical Oncology. 2013;**39**(5):482. DOI: 10.1016/j.ejso.2013.01.109

[56] Rezai M, Strauss S, Kimmig R, et al. Risk-reducing, conservative

mastectomy—Analysis of surgical outcome and quality of life in 272 implant-based reconstructions using TiLoop® bra versus autologous corial flaps. Gland Surgery. 2016;**5**(1):1-8. DOI: 10.3978/j.issn.2227-684X.2015.07.03

[57] Paepke S, Klein E, Kiechle M, et al. Implant-based mesh supported breast reconstruction: Patient reported outcome data (PRO-BRA trial, TiLOOP® bra) and perspectives. European Journal of Cancer. 2018;**92**(3):S87

[58] Caldon L, Allison C, Cain H, et al. The use of titanium mesh (TiLOOP) in immediate breast reconstruction; low cost, low complications. European Journal of Surgical Oncology. 2015;**41**(6):S69-S70. DOI: 10.1016/j.ejso.2015.03.193

[59] Eichler C, Schulz C, Thangarajah F, et al. A retrospective head-to-head comparison between TiLoop bra/TiMesh® and Seragyn® in 320 cases of reconstructive breast surgery. Anticancer Research. 2019;**39**(5):2599-2605. DOI: 10.21873/anticanres.13383

[60] Machleidt A, Schmidt-Feuerheerd N, Blohmer JU, et al. Reconstructive breast surgery with partially absorbable bi-component Seragyn® BR soft mesh: An outcome analysis. Archives of Gynecology and Obstetrics. 2018;**298**(4):755-761. DOI: 10.1007/s00404-018-4859-5

[61] Baldelli I, Cardoni G, Franchelli S, et al. Implant-based breast reconstruction using a polyester mesh (Surgimesh-PET): A retrospective single-center study. Plastic and Reconstructive Surgery. 2016;**137**(6):931e-939e. DOI: 10.1097/PRS.0000000000002180

[62] Rietgens M, De Lorenzi F, Venturino M, et al. The suspension technique to avoid the use of tissue expanders in breast reconstruction. Annals of Plastic Surgery. 2005;**54**:467-470. DOI: 10.1097/01.sap.0000155283.77188.63

[63] Sukhotko A, Zikiryahodjaev AD, Ermoshchenkova MV, et al. Implant-based breast cancer reconstruction with biological matric or synthetic mesh. Annals of Oncology. 2019;**30**(3):iii44

[64] Paepke S, Kiechle M, Ankel C, et al. Surgical studies of reconstructive breast surgery—An overview of the topics at the 2019 annual meeting of theWorking Group for Reconstructive Surgery in oncology-gynecology. Geburtshilfe und Frauenheilkunde. 2019;**79**:584-590

[65] Momoh AO, Ahmed R, Kelley BP, et al. A systematic review of complications of implant-based breast reconstruction with pre-reconstruction and post-reconstruction radiation therapy. Annals of Surgical Oncology. 2014;**21**(1):118-124. DOI: 10.1245/s10434-013-3284-z

[66] Nahabedian MY. AlloDerm performance in the setting of prosthetic breast surgery, infection, and irradiation. Plastic and Reconstructive Surgery. 2009;**124**(6):1743-1753

[67] Rawlani V, Buck DW 2nd, Johnson SA, et al. Tissue expander breast reconstruction using prehydrated human acellular dermis. Annals of Plastic Surgery. 2011;**66**(6):593-597

[68] Chun YS, Verma K, Rosen H, et al. Implant-based breast reconstruction using acellular dermal matrix and the risk of postoperative complications. Plastic and Reconstructive Surgery. 2010;**125**(2):429-436

[69] Moyer HR, Pinell-White X, Losken A. The effect of radiation on acellular dermal matrix and capsule formation in breast reconstruction: Clinical outcomes and histologic analysis. Plastic and Reconstructive Surgery. 2014;**133**:214-221

[70] Seth AK, Hirsch EM, Fine NA, et al. Utility of acellular dermis-assisted breast reconstruction in the setting of radiation: A comparative analysis. Plastic and Reconstructive Surgery. 2012;**130**:750-758

[71] Mylvaganam S, Conroy E, Williamson PR, et al. Variation in the provision and practice of implant-based breast reconstruction in the UK: Results from the iBRA national practice questionnaire. Breast. 2017;**35**:182-190. DOI: 10.1016/j.breast.2017.07.016

Chapter 10

L-Shaped Nipple Reconstruction: A Novel Technique to Improve Patient Satisfaction Outcomes

Krishnamurthy Sreedhar Murthy

Abstract

Nipple reconstruction is the final stage of breast reconstruction and performed after acceptable breast mound shape and symmetry has been achieved. The objectives of this study are to describe an original technique of nipple reconstruction, using a combination of random flap (for new nipple) and dermal graft (for new areola), and also measure patient satisfaction outcomes. Thirty-one patients underwent the L-shaped nipple reconstruction (2011-2016) at Liverpool Breast Unit and completed satisfaction survey of this technique. This cohort was compared to 59 patients who underwent traditional CV flap during the same period, in our Breast Unit. The study analysed the combined data of 90 patients (L flap N = 31 and CV flap N = 59). "L"-shaped flap is a random local skin flap to create new nipple and dermal graft is used to create new areola. There was no statistically significant difference in complication rates between traditional CV flap (9.7%) and L-shaped (13.6%) nipple reconstructions (Fishers exact test p = 0.74). In our L flap cohort, 94% were pleased and 93% would recommend it to a friend. Thus L flap is a viable alternative to CV flap in suitable patients and has positive patient satisfaction outcomes.

Keywords: L flap, nipple reconstruction, novel technique, patient satisfaction, areolar graft

1. Introduction

Reconstruction of nipple-areolar complex has been shown to have a positive influence on the overall recovery process of women undergoing post mastectomy breast reconstruction and hence helps to restore body image more completely. This clearly underscores the well-known concept that, part of the reconstruction of an aesthetically pleasing breast, is a high-quality nipple-areolar reconstruction [1].

Over the last 30 years, many different techniques have been described to accomplish this task. The goals for this nipple-areola reconstruction include appropriate nipple projection, areolar colour, and areolar texture. A number of reconstructive techniques have been described for nipple reconstruction including skin grafts, composite grafts, and various local flaps. Numerous techniques, using a variety of geometric designs, have been reported and reviewed [2–9]. Each of these techniques aims to achieve a natural shape with maintenance of projection over time, and minimal donor site morbidity. The most popular techniques benefit from simplicity, reliability and reproducibility.

Presented in this article is an original and novel technique, L shaped nipple reconstruction; which achieves these goals by providing an alternative to traditional techniques such as CV flap [9]. This has proven to be a suitable alternative option when previous mastectomy scars preclude optimum nipple positioning.

In this chapter, we share our institution's experience with the L flap nipple areolar reconstruction. Here, an earnest attempt is made to describe the indications for its use, flap design and surgical technique, and outcomes and complications associated with its use.

2. Patients and methods

Thirty-one patients underwent L shaped nipple reconstruction following breast reconstruction between 2011 and 2016, at Liverpool Breast Unit, Linda McCartney Centre. The study cohort were identified from prospectively collected data and analysed. All patients with transversely placed mastectomy scar, considered otherwise unsuitable for traditional CV flap reconstruction, were included in this study.

Once the patients were identified, their case notes were reviewed to record patient's age, body mass index, and position of previous mastectomy scar, type of breast reconstruction, chemotherapy, medical history, and smoking history. Complications explored included haematoma, postoperative wound healing problems, nipple-areola complex necrosis (partial and complete), infection, discharge, pain, fat necrosis and hypertrophic scarring.

Of the 31 patients, 17 patients (55%) had implant based reconstruction and 12 patients (39%) had latissimus dorsi (LD) with implant reconstruction and 2 patients (6%) had LD flap autologous breast shape reconstruction.

The timing of L flap reconstruction ranged from 6 months to 2 years after their initial cancer surgery or breast reconstruction, with an average time of 15 months.

Each patient was sent an outcome questionnaire, using validated Likert scoring scales (scale of 1–5), relating specifically to their nipple reconstruction. The questionnaire using Likert Scales was developed to evaluate overall patient satisfaction with cosmetic result, and addressed key issues, such as perceived match to contralateral nipple, confidence in clothing and reported complications.

3. Surgical technique

L-flap nipple reconstruction is a random skin flap, containing dermal and adipose tissue. It has a pedicle with long and short arms which resemble the letter L and hence the terminology. The L-flap was used on all our patients with transverse mastectomy scars, which would otherwise preclude the use of traditional flap, such as CV flap (**Figure 1**).

The traditional CV flap marked in **Figure 1**, would produce unsatisfactory neo-nipple position, i.e., above or below the mastectomy scar. Whereas, the alternate L shaped flap offers optimal neo-nipple position.

Preoperative marking was performed with patient standing to achieve ideal and closest natural nipple position. Marking with patient stood up would further ensure to centre the nipple symmetrically to the opposite side (natural or reconstructed nipple). The important markings included the patient's breast meridian, inframammary fold, and new nipple-areolar position (**Figure 2**).

The skin incision is made using no. 11 blade with depth of incision extending to pectoral fascia or onto subcutaneous tissue in event of autologous tissue breast shape reconstruction (**Figure 3**). The base of the L pedicle is measured to be equal to the nipple diameter to be created. The short arm lies opposite to the pedicle

(**Figure 3**). The long arm of the L flap is based on a laterally based random flap and is one and half to two times the diameter of the nipple. The marked long arm is raised and rotated through 180°, and sutured (**Figure 4**) with absorbable 4–0 monocryl (poliglecaprone 25, Ethicon) sutures. The short arm is then sutured to the upper border of long arm to create the summit of the neo-nipple and hence fashioned to create a projecting neo-nipple (**Figure 4**).

The area surrounding the reconstructed nipple site is de-epithelialised to match the areola on the native breast and this forms the first step in preparing the areolar base (**Figure 5**).

The next step involves harvesting and preparing the areolar graft from abdomen or from skin envelope of the opposite breast. The skin graft is then fashioned and placed over the raw surface to reconstruct the neo-areola (**Figure 6**), using absorbable 4–0 monocryl.

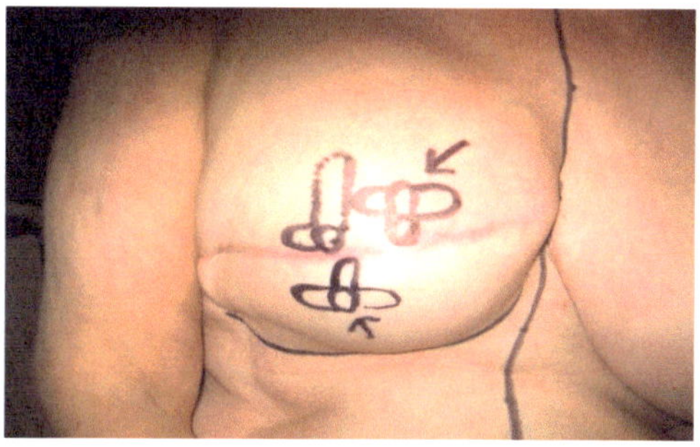

Figure 1.
Transverse mastectomy scar with mark up of L flap and CV flap (depicted with arrows).

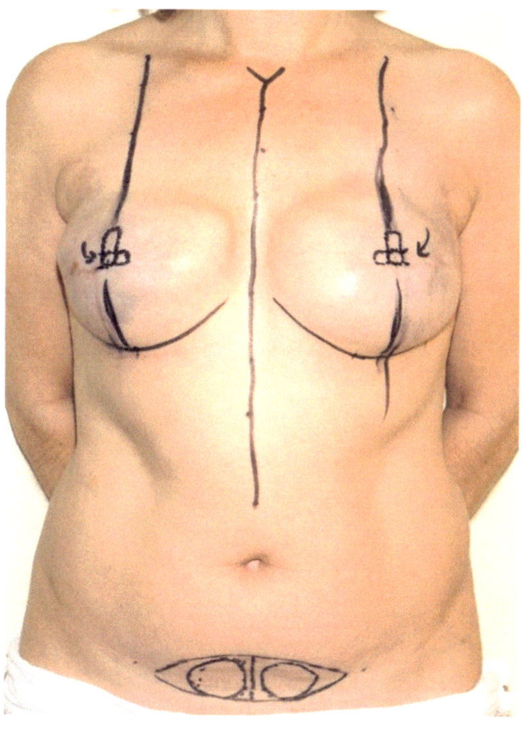

Figure 2.
Pre-operative markings for L flap nipple and areola.

The full thickness graft is fenestrated to facilitate drainage of serous collection or blood, which would ensure very low infection rates. The additional value of designing small openings in the graft is that it eventually generates the appearance of Montgomery tubercles over the neo-areola (**Figure** 7).

An interrupted 4–0 monocryl suture is used to secure the skin to the graft. Once the graft is secured, the entire neo-nipple/areolar complex is covered with Mepitel or Jelonet, covered with surgical gauze with a central button hole; all held together with clear Tegaderm hydrocolloid dressings. Tegaderm backing allows the patient to shower, easy to use and can be applied one-handed. The dressing is left intact for

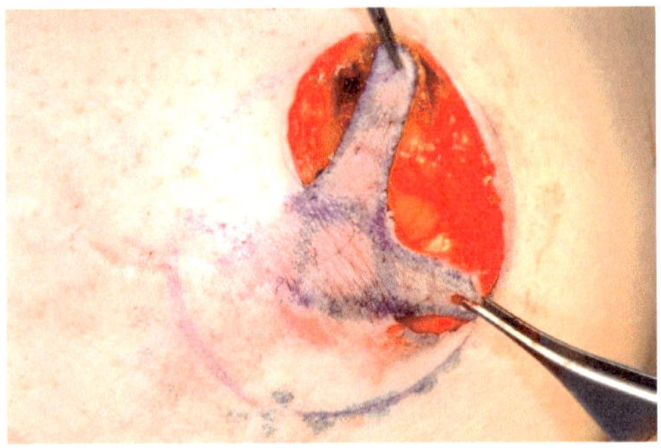

Figure 3.
Details of raising the L flap.

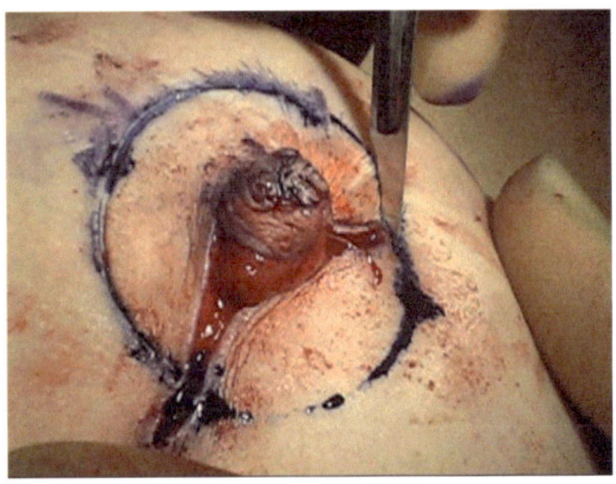

Figure 4.
Neo-nipple inset and creation of base for areola.

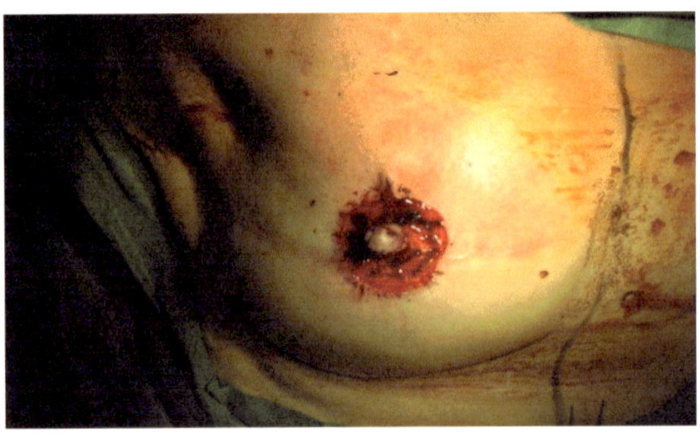

Figure 5.
De-epithelialised neo-areolar base.

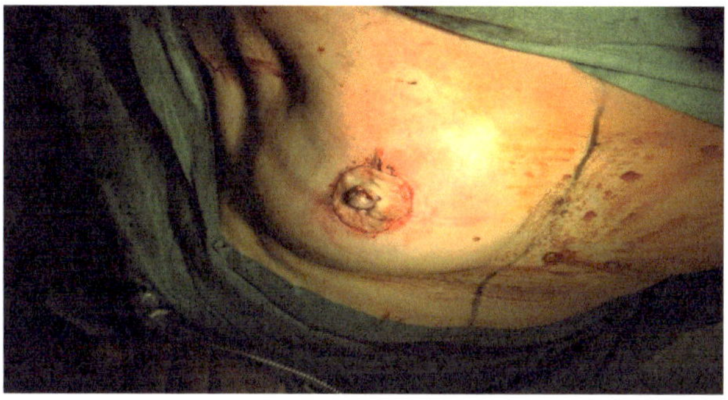

Figure 6.
Full thickness skin graft to create neo-areola.

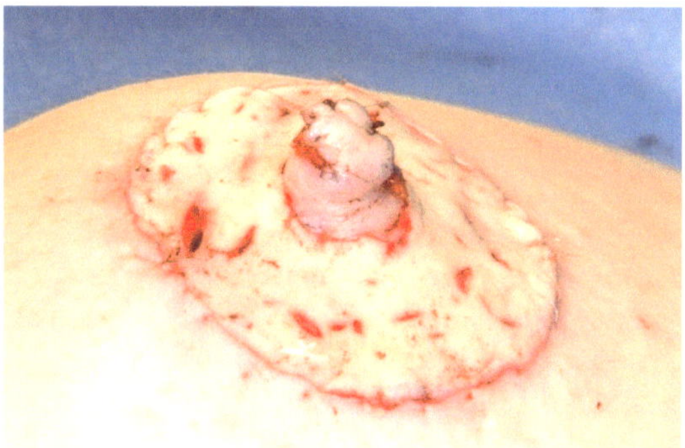

Figure 7.
A per op view of neo-nipple and neo-areola with typical fenestrations.

10 days until the outpatient clinic review, wherein all 31 patients were reviewed by the Surgeon.

Prophylactic antibiotics are administered, with Co-amoxiclav (500 mg/125 mg) being our antibiotic of choice. In patients with allergies to penicillin, we found macrolide antibiotics such as erythromycin or clarithromycin helpful.

4. Statistical analysis

The data of complications from concurrently performed traditional CV flap was compared with the novel L-flap technique.

The categorical data were summarised using frequencies, percentages, cross tabulation and bar chart and analysed by Fisher's exact test. All statistics and analyses were produced using IBM SPSS version 20.

5. Results

A total of 31 patients met inclusion criteria (previous transverse mastectomy scar and not deemed suitable for CV flap nipple-areola reconstruction) and were evaluated. The mean age of patients identified was 44 years (range, 33–64 years) and the mean body mass index was 28 (range, 24–32). Patients displayed minimal medical co-morbidities, and there were no patients who were actively smoking at the time of surgery.

All patients had undergone total mastectomy and had well healed transversely placed chest wall scars. Twelve patients (38.7%) were treated with chemotherapy (Adriamycin with or without Paclitaxel) and none of the 31 patients underwent external beam irradiation.

Intra-operatively, all patients underwent L-shaped flap nipple reconstruction with areolar skin graft from abdomen or contralateral breast, with technique as described above.

As depicted in **Table 1**; the incidence of any complications, including infection, discharge, pain, bleeding, partial or total nipple loss; as compared with traditional CV flap were similar and no statistically significant difference (Fisher's exact test).

Table 2 summarises the patients' undergoing L flap showed good cosmetic outcomes in comparison with patients' undergoing CV flap in the same breast Unit during the same period of time as the study cohort.

Table 3 shows that nipple projection in the study cohort of L flap compared favourably with patients' undergoing traditional CV flap, over 6 and 24 months.

6. Discussion

Nipple reconstruction and patient satisfaction outcomes study seem to be an area of very limited research and hence lack of evidence based scientific literature. While nipple reconstruction is considered a minor procedure, its profound implications on patient satisfaction after post-mastectomy breast reconstruction have been clearly demonstrated [9, 10].

Complications	L flap (n = 31)	CV flap (n = 59)	P-value (Fisher's exact test)
Superficial nipple tip necrosis	3 (10%)	6 (10%)	P = 1.0
Cellulitis	2 (6%)	3 (5%)	P = 1.0
Pain	2 (6%)	5 (8%)	P = 1.0
Bleeding/haematoma	1 (3%)	3 (5%)	P = 1.0
Partial nipple loss	2 (6%)	2 (3%)	P = 0.60
Surgical revision	2 (6%)	3 (5%)	P = 1.0

Table 1.
Complications: L flap and CV flap nipple reconstructions compared.

	L flap (n = 31)	CV flap (n = 59)	P-value
Overall cosmetic outcome—satisfied/very satisfied	90% (n = 28)	86% (n = 51)	P = 0.74
Wearing daily clothes—confident/very confident	81% (n = 25)	69% (n = 41)	P = 0.32
Wearing swim clothes—confident/very confident	77% (n = 24)	63% (n = 37)	P = 0.24
Wearing night clothes—confident/very confident	71% (n = 22)	63% (n = 37)	P = 0.49
Nipple Reconstruction-Good/Very Good Match to opposite side	77%(n = 24)	69%(n = 41)	P = 0.47

Table 2.
PROMs (patient reported outcome measures) in each of the techniques.

Nipple projection	L flap	CV flap
Immediate post-op	4–5 mm (4.5 mm)	5–6 mm (5.5 mm)
6 months follow-up	3–5 mm (4 mm)	4–5 mm (4.5 mm)
24 months follow-up	2–4 mm (3 mm)	2–4 mm (3 mm)

Table 3.
Comparison of nipple projection between two cohorts.

A vast majority of contributions related to nipple reconstruction merely focus on surgical techniques. Literature review has shown a major emphasis of articles has been on ways to prevent the inevitable loss of nipple projection [11–16]. This is in contrast to the limited number of studies analysing risk factors and complication rates after nipple reconstruction [13, 17].

It is prudent, however, to not only concentrate on preservation of nipple projection but also analyse and identify factors that predict poor outcome, as complications after nipple reconstruction can have devastating consequences for patients.

It is reasonable for the patient undergoing breast shape reconstruction to expect the same high standards of nipple-areolar reconstruction as the breast mound itself [18]. Hence it would be prudent to give the greatest consideration to the position of the new nipple-areola complex and to the symmetry on the other side. It is important to assert that nipple-areola reconstruction represents the final stage of breast reconstruction, whereby a reconstructed breast mound is transformed into a breast facsimile that more closely resembles the original breast. Shestak et al. in their salient review of Assessment of Long-Term Nipple Projection—A Comparison of Three Techniques, using either a bell flap, a modified star flap, or a skate flap and full-thickness skin graft for areola reconstruction; note that loss of nipple and areola projection was quite remarkable using the bell flap and hence would discourage its use in virtually all patients requiring nipple-areola reconstructions [19]. They find the other two techniques reviewed, i.e., modified star flap and skate flap with full-thickness skin graft for areolar reconstruction, to be more suitable in a variety of situations to maintain long term nipple projections [19].

The complexity and outcomes of the creation of a new nipple areola following cancer surgery is succinctly demonstrated by Sisti et al. [20] In their seminal review of literature, the authors having thoroughly analysed 75 papers published over 69 years, and have observed that flaps have held the "*test of time*" in nipple reconstructions. Overcorrection of nipple projection (up to 50%), in suitable patients, to prevent long term loss of nipple projection is an interesting observation in this review. In this context, being informed and sharing decision making with patients, helps patient empowerment and improves overall satisfaction. This concept could support future studies involving techniques, outcomes and influence patient confidence which would all further enhance patient safety.

This novel L-flap nipple reconstruction was devised and developed at Liverpool Breast Unit, to provide a viable and robust alternative to traditional flaps and keeping with patient's expectations and interest. This technique seems a very useful resource considering several criteria it should fulfil to near match contralateral native nipple areolar complex or a previously reconstructed neo-nipple. Our clinical observation over the years of an unsatisfactory nipple position with traditional CV flap, in people with transversely placed mastectomy scar, has led us to develop this innovative L flap. The outcomes of PROMs (patient reported outcome measures), in addition to our clinical observation of a better and satisfactory nipple position achieved with L flap have supported our journey to develop this L flap.

Our choice of creating neo-areola by means of a full-thickness graft has resulted in a better colour match and projection compared with other techniques, such as tattooing.

In this study we have noted complication rates in all our L-shaped flaps are not significantly different from the traditional and well established CV flap. There was no statistically significant difference in complication rates between both types of nipple reconstruction, although perceived clinical difference should be individually addressed. These outcomes support our nascent work of developing a technique to enhance patient satisfaction.

We acknowledge the study limitations being small population sizes and intermediate follow up period. A larger group of patients and a longer follow up will help us draw conclusions, with particular attention to nipple projection. Analysing the patient feedback and reflecting on the overall outcomes, we are pleased that we have developed and presented a novel technique to enhance patient care and safety. This provides further stimulus to our on-going service improvement project keeping In line with modern National Health Services, "patient centred care".

7. Conclusions

This novel design for nipple-areola complex reconstruction can be used in either primary or secondary nipple reconstruction. Of particular and distinct advantage is that all the scars are contained within the peripheral peri-areolar incision and thus can be completely camouflaged by an intra-dermal tattoo. Nipple projection has been consistently maintained and outcomes are reasonable and are similar to that of a CV flap. The creative use of patient's own tissue expands the utility of the L flap beyond its current application in poorly placed transverse mastectomy scars.

Acknowledgements

We acknowledge Dr. Poornima Murthy BDS, MPH, FRSH, for her help in manuscript preparation and graphics.

We would like to thank Mr. M.V. Chandrashekar for sharing the pictures of L flap nipple reconstruction.

Conflict of interest statement

None.

Funding

None.

Author details

Krishnamurthy Sreedhar Murthy
National Health Services, United Kingdom

*Address all correspondence to: rksmurthy@gmail.com

References

[1] Bogue DP, Mungara AK, Thompson M, Cederna PS. Modified technique for nipple-areolar reconstruction: A case series. Plastic & Reconstructive Surgery. 2003;**112**(5):1274-1278

[2] Farhadi J, Maksvytyte GK, Schaefer DJ, Pierer G, Scheufler O. Reconstruction of the nipple-areola complex: An update. Journal of Plastic, Reconstructive & Aesthetic Surgery. 2006;**59**:40-53

[3] Shestak KC, Nguyen TD. The double opposing periareola flap: A novel concept for nipple-areola reconstruction. Plastic and Reconstructive Surgery. 2007;**119**:473-480

[4] Eo S, Kim SS, Da Lio AL. Nipple reconstruction with C-V flap using dermofat graft. Annals of Plastic Surgery. 2007;**58**:137-140

[5] Schoeller T, Schubert HM, Pulzl P, et al. Nipple reconstruction using a modified arrow flap technique. Breast. 2006;**15**:762-768

[6] Germano D, De Biasio F, Piedimonte A, et al. Nipple reconstruction using the fleur-de-lis flap technique. Aesthetic Plastic Surgery. 2006;**30**:399-402

[7] Gamboa-Bobadilla GM. Nipple reconstruction: The top hat technique. Annals of Plastic Surgery. 2005;**54**:243-246

[8] Rubino C, Dessy LA, Posadinu A. A modified technique for nipple reconstruction: The 'arrow flap'. British Journal of Plastic Surgery. 2003;**56**:247-251

[9] Losken A, Mackay GJ, Bastwick J. Nipple reconstruction using C-V flap technique: A long-term evaluation. Plastic and Reconstructive Surgery. 2001;**108**:361

[10] Shaikh-Naidu N, Preminger BA, Rogers K, Messina P, Gayle LB. Determinants of aesthetic satisfaction following TRAM and implant breast reconstruction. Annals of Plastic Surgery. 2004;**52**:465-470. Discussion 470

[11] Shestak KC, Gabriel A, Landecker A, Peters S, Shestak A, Kim J. Assessment of long-term nipple projection: A comparison of three techniques. Plastic and Reconstructive Surgery. 2002;**110**:780-786

[12] Shestak KC, Nguyen TD. The double opposing periareola flap: A novel concept for nipple-areola reconstruction. Plastic and Reconstructive Surgery. 2007;**119**:473-480

[13] Zhong T, Antony A, Cordeiro P. Surgical outcomes and nipple projection using the modified skate flap for nipple-areolar reconstruction in a series of 422 implant reconstructions. Annals of Plastic Surgery. 2009;**62**:591-595

[14] Rosing JH, Momeni A, Kamperman K, Kahn D, Gurtner G, Lee GK. Effectiveness of the Asteame nipple guard (TM) in maintaining projection following nipple reconstruction: A prospective randomised controlled trial. Journal of Plastic, Reconstructive & Aesthetic Surgery. 2010;**63**(10):1592-1596

[15] Eo S, Kim SS, Da Lio AL. Nipple reconstruction with C-V flap using dermofat graft. Annals of Plastic Surgery. 2007;**58**:137-140

[16] Jones AP, Erdmann M. Projection and patient satisfaction using the "hamburger" nipple reconstruction technique. Journal of Plastic,

Reconstructive & Aesthetic Surgery. 2012;**65**:207-212

[17] Draper LB, Bui DT, Chiu ES, et al. Nipple-areola reconstruction following chest-wall irradiation for breast cancer: Is it safe? Annals of Plastic Surgery. 2005;**55**:12-15

[18] Little JW III. Nipple-areola reconstruction. Plastic & Reconstructive Surgery. November 1985;**76**(5):806

[19] Shestak KC, Gabriel A, Landecker A, Peters S, Shestak A, Kim J. Assessment of long-term nipple projection: A comparison of three techniques. Plastic and Reconstructive Surgery. 2002;**110**:780

[20] Sisti A, Grimaldi L, Tassinari J, Cuomo R, Fortezza L, Bocchiotti MA, et al. Nipple-areola complex reconstruction techniques: A literature review. European Journal of Surgical Oncology. 2016 Apr;**42**(4):441-465